Mrs. Hendrix
It is a p'
to help care'
keep up the "pace!"

Best
Jeff

WHAT ARE

Palpitations

AND ABNORMAL HEART RHYTHMS (ARRHYTHMIAS)?

A CARDIOLOGIST'S GUIDE FOR PATIENTS AND CARE PROVIDERS

Dr. Jeffrey L. Williams

ISBN: 0692904212
ISBN-13: 9780692904213
Library of Congress Control Number: 2017909335
Cardiologist's Guides, Lebanon, PA

To my wife and three great kids for giving this life meaning.

To my patients for, well…tolerating me.

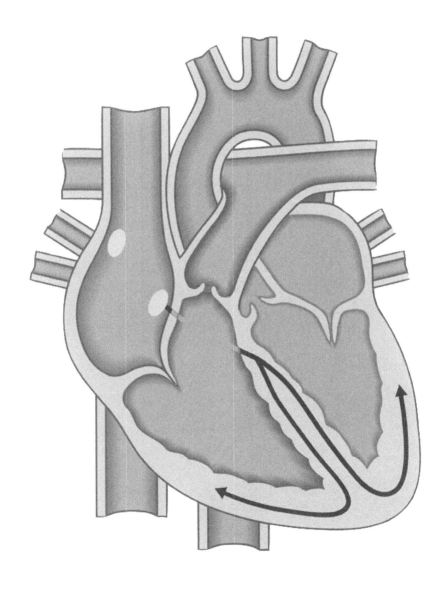

Contents

List of Figures

List of Tables

Introduction

The hectic pace at which today's doctors conduct their practices has shortchanged the information-sharing process for patients, especially those undergoing evaluation for heart-rhythm disorders. Patients and their families are often unaware of many critical issues involved in diagnosing and treating heart-rhythm disorders. Any treatment plan entails risks that are particular for each patient, medication, and procedure. I have found it increasingly difficult to provide a complete consultation, physical exam, and discussion about the risks and benefits of and alternatives to heart-rhythm treatment in a typical forty-five-minute session. Since starting a Heart Rhythm Center in 2008, I have developed several iterations of written and online patient-education materials to complement our office discussions. This book serves as a comprehensive summary of the steps involved in heart-rhythm evaluation, from the initial assessment and treatment to the possible performance of an invasive electrophysiology study (and possible ablation) and the required long-term follow-up care for patients and their caregivers (both professional and laypeople alike). Furthermore, because many of my patients (young and old) rely on their spouses and families for help with the decision-making process and long-term care of their heart-rhythm abnormalities, this book serves as a thorough means to ensure that all family members understand the types of arrhythmias that may be encountered and the treatment options that are available.

Palpitations are the sensation of an irregular, fast, uncomfortable, or strong heartbeat. Over six hundred thousand patients present to emergency departments each year in the United States (Probst et al. 2014) because of palpitations. One in four of these patients will be admitted to the hospital for further care, and roughly a third of patients will be diagnosed with a heart condition.

This book is dedicated solely to patients, families, and other care providers as a comprehensive review of the "what, why, and how" of palpitations and heart-rhythm abnormalities. As patients become more and more invested in decisions that affect their health care, they need more detailed information in order to make comprehensive assessments before deciding on the most appropriate treatment for their particular condition. This book can be part of the informed-consent process because it covers all aspects of abnormal heart-rhythm evaluation in a more thorough manner than can be presented in a single office visit or even multiple visits. Chapter 1 offers very detailed discussions about heart function—I've tried not to overwhelm the reader but felt that I needed to include advanced information for readers who would like this level of detail. In later chapters, particular emphasis is placed on the types of arrhythmias, why they may occur, and the treatment options available. If you don't understand some of the words in this text, there is a full glossary at the end of the book. Ultimately, patients who are concerned that they may have a heart-rhythm abnormality will find this book a useful summary of the complete evaluation that is performed.

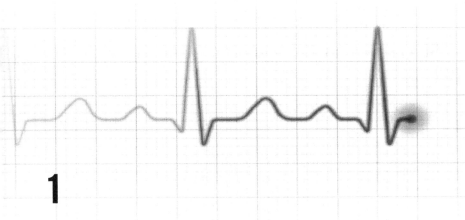

1

Basics of Heart Anatomy and the Conduction System

Blood flow through the heart. Figure 1 depicts the basic structure of the heart. Blood returns from the body and enters the right atrium. The blood leaves the right atrium through the tricuspid valve and enters the right ventricle. The right ventricle then pumps the blood through the pulmonary valve into the lungs. The blood is oxygenated in the lungs and is returned to the left atrium. The blood leaves the left atrium through the mitral valve and enters the left ventricle. The left ventricle pumps the oxygenated blood through the aortic valve to the rest of the body; it then returns to the heart via the right atrium.

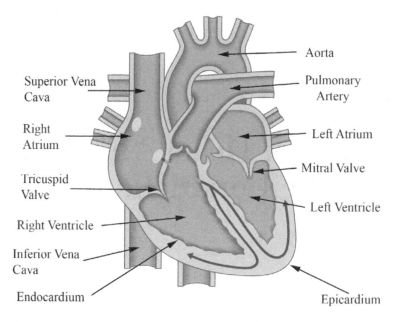

Figure 1. Basic Anatomy of the Heart

If the coronary arteries of the heart represent the "plumbing," then the conduction system of the heart represents the "wiring." Figure 2 presents the conduction system of the heart. A normal heart rate is sixty to one hundred beats per minute (bpm). *Bradycardia* is an abnormally slow heart rate, less than 60 bpm, and *tachycardia* refers to an abnormally fast heart rate, greater than 100 bpm. The sinoatrial (SA) node serves as the internal clock—or natural pacemaker—of the heart and signals the appropriate heart rate for a given situation.

Electrical conduction system of the heart. The heart's natural pacemaker (the SA node) is located in the top-right chamber of the heart: the right atrium. The SA node sends a signal to the upper chambers (the right and left atria) and the lower chambers (the right and left ventricles) via the atrioventricular (AV) node. The AV node transmits the electrical signal to the bottom chambers via the left and right bundle branches. The left bundle branch is composed of left-posterior and left-anterior *fascicles*, another term for divisions or branches. Often, the patient has a slow heart rate because the electrical connection between the top (the signal from the SA node) and bottom (the ventricles) of the heart is impaired; this condition is called an *AV block*. The most common type of pacemaker involves placing leads in the right atrium and right ventricle if we are treating AV block that is causing worrisome symptoms.

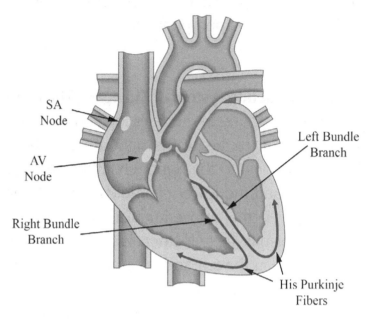

Figure 2. Conduction System of the Heart

Coronary arteries. The coronary arteries supply blood (and hence, oxygen) to the heart muscle; they course along the outside of the heart (*epicardium*). Each coronary artery supplies particular muscle territories in the heart. The left main coronary artery comes off the aorta and branches into the left-anterior descending (LAD) and circumflex (CX) arteries. The right coronary artery (RCA) comes off the right side of the aorta and ultimately branches into the posterolateral (PLA) and posterior descending arteries (PDA). See table 1 for the blood supplies of various elements of the conduction system. An AV block is often seen during heart attacks (blockages of coronary arteries) involving the RCA because in 80 percent of patients, the AV-node blood supply is provided by the RCA. In addition, a left-posterior fascicular block is uncommonly due to coronary disease because it has a dual blood supply. It would require two occluded coronary arteries (PDA and LAD septal perforators) to become blocked.

Table 1. Blood Supply to the Heart's Electrical Conduction System

Structure	Blood Supply
SA Node	55% RCA; 35% Left Circumflex; 10% Dual
AV Node	80% RCA; 10% Left Circumflex; 10% Dual
RBB	LAD Septal Perforators, AV Nodal Branch of RCA
LBB: LAF	LAD Septal Perforators
LBB: LPF	PDA and LAD Septal Perforators

SA=sinoatrial, AV=atrioventricular, RBB=right bundle branch, LBB=left bundle branch, LAF=left-anterior fascicle, LPF=left-posterior fascicle.

Electrocardiogram (ECG or EKG). One of the most important tools that doctors have to assess the electrical function of your heart is the electrocardiogram. Figure 3 depicts a typical electrocardiogram tracing and shows how this waveform represents the electrical and pumping actions of your heart. A typical ECG in your doctor's office has twelve leads (or tracings) because this allows your doctor to better localize arrhythmias and areas of prior heart attacks as well as other structural abnormalities.

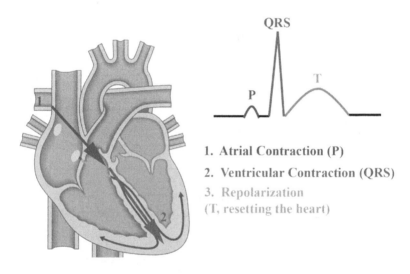

1. Atrial Contraction (P)
2. Ventricular Contraction (QRS)
3. Repolarization
(T, resetting the heart)

Figure 3. The Electrocardiogram and Its Relation to Heart Timing/ Pumping

The *P wave* corresponds to the electrical activation of the right and left atria. The right and left atria contract and pump the blood to the right and left ventricles, respectively. The *PR interval* is the time it takes for electrical activation from the SA node through the AV node to the right and left ventricles. The PR interval is measured from the beginning of the P wave to the onset of the QRS complex. The *QRS complex* is the electrical representation of the right and left ventricles contracting and pumping blood out of the heart. The *T wave* corresponds to repolarization (or resetting of the ventricles' electrical system) prior to the next contraction of the heart. The time from the onset of the QRS complex to the end of the T wave (called the *QT interval*) can be prolonged in patients at risk for sudden cardiac death. *An **arrhythmia** is a disruption of this orderly progression of SA-node activation through the AV node and the right and left ventricles (via the His-Purkinje system which carries the electrical impulse from the right and left bundle branches to the muscle of the right and left ventricles).*

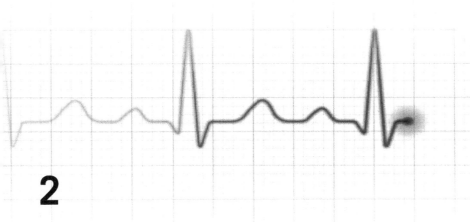

2

Palpitations and Other Symptoms That May Represent Heart-Rhythm Abnormalities (Arrhythmias)

Introduction. Heart-rhythm abnormalities are actually quite common, and thankfully, the majority are not life threatening. Figure 4A shows the incidence of arrhythmias in adults. Arrhythmias generally do not occur as frequently in younger patients. These different types of arrhythmias are discussed in chapters 5, 6, and 7.

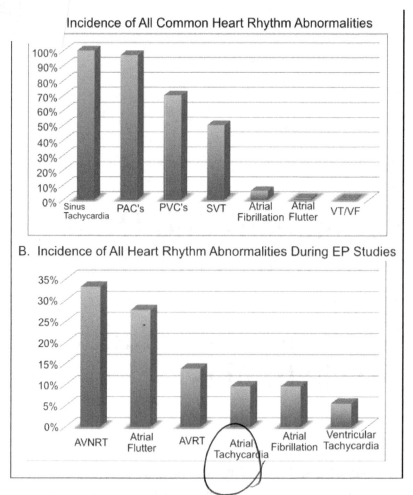

Figure 4. Common Heart-Rhythm Disorders Seen in Adults and the Electrophysiology (EP) Laboratory. Panel A shows the incidence (percentage of total patients) of heart-rhythm disorders in all adults. Panel B shows the incidence of arrhythmias in patients undergoing EP studies with ablations during a typical year of practice in a community hospital EP program. One can see that some heart-rhythm abnormalities, such as sinus tachycardia (the fast heart rhythm during exercise), occur in almost everyone. PAC=premature atrial contraction, PVC=premature ventricular contraction, SVT=supraventricular tachycardia, VT=ventricular tachycardia, VF=ventricular fibrillation, AVNRT= atrioventricular nodal reentrant tachycardia, AVRT=atrioventricular reentrant tachycardia.

It is important to note that heart-rhythm problems can be quite common, but we must have an understanding of the difference between a normal and abnormal heart rhythm.

What is a normal heart rhythm? A normal heart rhythm is when your heart rate is between sixty and one hundred beats per minute (bpm), with one atrial and one ventricular contraction for each heartbeat. This is called normal sinus rhythm. As discussed in chapter 1, the sinus node is a specialized area in your heart that serves as the "timer" or "pacemaker" for your heart. Any heart rate above 100 bpm or below 60 bpm could be abnormal. However, there are some situations where a heart rate may be less than 60 bpm but not indicate an abnormality, such as in a well-trained athlete at rest; the most common situation is called *sinus bradycardia*, and no treatment is necessary. Similarly, there are some situations where a heart rate may be more than 100 bpm, such as during illness or infection; the most common explanation for this is called *sinus tachycardia*, and treatment of the underlying illness will correct the fast heart rhythm.

What are abnormal heart rhythms? Abnormal heart rhythms include a multitude of situations in which the heart rate is outside the normal range of 60 to

100 bpm. Furthermore, an abnormal heart rhythm can also occur within the normal range of between 60 and 100 bpm, and this is detected with a twelve-lead electrocardiogram. Another cause of abnormal heart rhythms is when the heart beats irregularly for any reason. Not all abnormal or irregular heart rhythms are worrisome or need treatment; however, this book discusses many of the common abnormal heart rhythms and the treatment options that are available.

What are palpitations? *Palpitations are the sensation of an irregular, fast, uncomfortable, or strong heartbeat.* These symptoms may be caused by an abnormal heart rhythm, but I have many patients with palpitations that are not associated with any arrhythmia. It is important to note that many patients will not experience palpitations but still have an arrhythmia. Finally, not all patients with "palpitations" have a heart-rhythm abnormality; this can be very frustrating for the patient, but we can at least offer reassurance that there is not an active cardiac issue.

Other symptoms that may represent heart-rhythm abnormalities. My goal as a care provider for heart-rhythm disorders is to carefully listen to the patient describing his or her symptoms and determine the likelihood that these symptoms may represent a heart-rhythm abnormality. Many patients who have an arrhythmia will not tell me that they are "having a fast heartbeat." Often, patients report fluttering, vibrating, skipping, or tingling. Furthermore, patients may not experience these symptoms in the chest but instead experience symptoms in the stomach, neck, jaw, or back. I have had a patient report belching; careful questioning revealed that the patient had a heart-rhythm abnormality that caused her to feel nauseous and start belching!

Know your ejection fraction. The best single predictor for risk of possibly harmful arrhythmias (and risk of sudden cardiac death) is your *ejection fraction*, which refers to how much blood your heart pumps with every beat. The ejection fraction is most commonly measured during echocardiography (an ultrasound of your heart) or stress testing. Your ejection fraction may also be measured during a computed tomography (CT) scan or magnetic resonance imaging (MRI) of your heart. In addition, the multigated acquisition (MUGA) scan is a special test that can be used to measure your heart's ejection fraction. Talk to your care provider about the type of test used to measure your ejection fraction. The healthy heart ejects 55 to 70 percent of the blood it can hold during every beat. Once a patient's heart pumps less than 35 percent during a typical heartbeat, the patient is considered at risk for sudden cardiac death and may be a candidate for a defibrillator. It must be emphasized, however, that there are several situations in which a defibrillator is recommended if the ejection fraction is greater than 35 percent; these include hypertrophic cardiomyopathy, long-QT syndrome, and other situations that are outside the scope of this book.

What are ventricular fibrillation and ventricular tachycardia? *Ventricular tachycardia* refers to a very fast beating of the bottom chambers of the heart (the ventricles), and it can cause low blood pressure, loss of consciousness, and even death if not treated. *Ventricular fibrillation* refers to an even faster beating of the bottom chambers of the heart (the ventricles) and is often fatal. During *sudden cardiac death*, when the heart goes into ventricular fibrillation, the bottom chambers only quiver, and no blood is pumped. This leads to a loss of blood pressure, followed by loss of consciousness (called *syncope* or fainting) and then, if not stopped quickly, death. It may seem confusing, but it is possible to survive sudden cardiac death. A person can faint because of sudden cardiac death (i.e., ventricular fibrillation, as shown in figure 5) and be revived quickly, depending on the underlying medical condition and availability of emergency personnel.

Figure 5 shows the electrocardiogram of a patient who had an episode of ventricular fibrillation while hospitalized. This patient quickly underwent electrical *cardioversion* and had a defibrillator placed to stop further episodes of ventricular fibrillation. Cardioversion is a procedure using electricity (as in this case) or medicines to convert an abnormally fast heart rhythm to a normal rhythm.

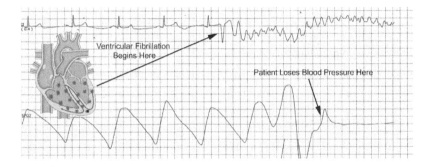

Figure 5. Ventricular Fibrillation Causing Cardiac Arrest

Is there a difference between atrial fibrillation and ventricular fibrillation? Atrial fibrillation and ventricular fibrillation are *very* different. Atrial fibrillation is the most common clinical arrhythmia encountered in cardiac electrophysiology, and it is a problem of the top chambers in your heart—that is, the atria. Approximately 5 percent of people over sixty years of age have this condition. If you have atrial fibrillation, your most significant risk is for stroke, and the first step in treatment is deciding what type of anticoagulation is appropriate for your situation. Aspirin alone may be adequate, but you may require warfarin or one of the newer oral anticoagulants that can be used in place of warfarin (e.g., Coumadin). The next issue is to determine how to manage the heart-rhythm abnormality itself. A *rhythm-control* strategy is in place when you are given *antiarrhythmics* (medications that help maintain a normal rhythm) to prevent atrial fibrillation from happening; this strategy is ideal for patients with severe symptoms. Antiarrhythmics include flecainide, propafenone, amiodarone, sotalol, dofetilide, and dronedarone. A *rate-control* strategy allows the presence of atrial fibrillation but prevents fast heart rates with medications to slow your heart rate; this is a good option for patients who do not feel their atrial fibrillation (three out of ten patients with atrial fibrillation may not have symptoms). Medications to help slow your heart while you are in atrial fibrillation include beta-blockers (e.g., metoprolol, atenolol, and carvedilol), calcium-channel blockers (e.g., diltiazem and verapamil), and digoxin.

The most important thing to realize is that atrial fibrillation will not be completely treated (or understood) in a single visit. Be patient with your care provider. A medicine that works for one patient may not work for another. Remember: atrial fibrillation is very different from ventricular fibrillation! See chapter 6 for more about atrial fibrillation.

Congestive heart failure and risk of arrhythmias. It is confusing, but congestive heart failure (CHF) may cause arrhythmias, and arrhythmias may be the cause of CHF. Symptoms of CHF may include the following:

- shortness of breath during exertion or while lying down
- chest pain
- swelling (edema) in the feet, ankles, or legs
- irregular or fast heart rate
- weakness and fatigue
- reduced ability to walk or exercise
- coughing (sometimes with pink sputum) or wheezing
- sudden weight gain
- loss of appetite or stomach discomfort

The appearance of these symptoms should be relayed to your doctor.

The American College of Cardiology has developed extensive guidelines for the diagnosis and treatment of heart failure (Hunt et al. 2001). A doctor who suspects heart failure may check your electrocardiogram, evaluate your blood laboratory tests (discussed in chapter 4), and assess your ejection fraction to find the underlying cause of the heart failure. Coronary-artery blockages are the underlying cause for two-thirds of patients with heart failure (called *ischemic cardiomyopathy*). The remaining patients have heart failure caused by arrhythmia, hypertension, heart-valve disease, heart-muscle (myocardial) disease, or toxins such as alcohol or some types of cancer medications. Sometimes, patients have no obvious cause for their heart failure (called *idiopathic cardiomyopathy*).

The true incidence of arrhythmias causing CHF is not clearly known but is probably underrecognized (Gopinathannair et al. 2015). Atrial fibrillation is an arrhythmia that is very common and is found in as many as 10 to 50 percent of patients with CHF. However, CHF is less commonly caused by arrhythmias; CHF caused by arrhythmia may occur in as few as one in ten patients with arrhythmias from the atrium and as many as one in three patients with arrhythmias from the ventricle. Obviously, arrhythmias in patients with CHF are generally more concerning than arrhythmias in patients with no evidence of CHF.

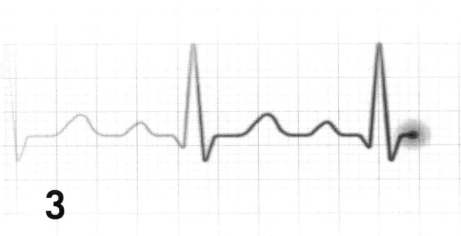

3

How Are Heart-Rhythm Abnormalities Diagnosed?

Introduction. Your care providers have extensive training in assessing the possible arrhythmias that may be causing your symptoms. There are different levels of training among primary care providers, cardiologists, and electrophysiologists (discussed in chapter 4); however, the diagnosis of abnormal heart rhythms can often be accomplished with some basic tests.

It must be noted that arrhythmias can be very tricky to diagnose, and sometimes, it is like taking your car to the mechanic; just like your car may not make "that noise" when the mechanic is under the hood, your heart may not have an abnormal rhythm when you are undergoing one of the tests discussed in this chapter. Be patient with your care providers, as I have had patients with palpitations where it took over thirty years to document their arrhythmias, which occurred at random times! My goal is to get a recording of your heart rhythm while you are having the concerning symptoms and document any arrhythmia if present. Once I can ascertain the particular arrhythmia causing your symptoms, it is easier to tailor the correct therapy to alleviate the symptoms. Additionally, symptoms sometimes are *not* due to an abnormal heart rhythm; this is also helpful because it allows your care providers to at least rule out a heart issue as a cause for your symptoms and look for other causes.

Electrocardiogram (ECG or EKG). One of the most important tools that doctors have to assess the electrical function of your heart is the electrocardiogram. Figure 3 in chapter 1 depicts a typical electrocardiogram tracing and shows how this waveform represents the electrical and pumping actions of your heart. A typical ECG in your doctor's office has twelve leads (or tracings) because this allows your doctor to better localize arrhythmias and areas of prior heart attacks as well as other structural abnormalities. We will go over the appearance of common ECGs during arrhythmias later in this book (see chapter 5, figure 7). The standard ECG only records ten seconds of your heart rhythm, so if your symptoms occur once or twice a day, it is unlikely we will be lucky enough to capture it with the ECG.

Twenty-four-hour Holter monitor. Oftentimes, *for symptoms that occur daily, the first test we will obtain is a Holter monitor.* This involves several electrodes (patches that are temporarily taped to your skin) that are worn for twenty-four to forty-eight hours. The monitor is applied in the office and is worn home. The more consistently it is worn, the more thorough the ability to look for arrhythmia. It is generally taken off for showers; however, there are some systems that can be worn while showering. Please check with your care provider before getting any of these devices wet because they are very expensive to replace (e.g., "you break it, you buy it!"). The Holter monitor will continuously record your heart rhythm while it is worn. Once the set time period for wearing device is met, the Holter is brought back to the office, where we examine the recordings for any arrhythmia. A paper diary is usually provided with the monitor so that you can write down the time a particular symptom is experienced to help correlate any symptoms with your heart rhythm.

Two- to four-week outpatient telemetry monitor. The telemetry monitor involves similar skin patches as used in a Holter, but it continuously monitors your heart rhythm for two to four weeks at a time. *These are best suited for symptoms that may only occur once or twice a week.* Like the Holter monitor, it is applied in the office and worn home. Generally, it is taken off for showers. These devices also have the ability to allow a patient to "activate" a recording when any symptom is felt that might represent an abnormal heart rhythm. Once the set time period has been met, the device is brought (or even mailed) back to the office, where we can analyze the recordings for arrhythmia. Another name for this is mobile cardiac outpatient telemetry (MCOT).

Hospital telemetry. Many patients are admitted to the hospital and are placed on *telemetry*. Telemetry is a system that utilizes skin patches that continuously record your heart rhythm and automatically send reports to the hospital nursing stations. These reports can often document arrhythmias, and they will be examined by the professionals caring for you in the hospital. A common reason I am asked to evaluate a patient is when an abnormal heart rhythm is discovered while the patient is being monitored on telemetry while hospitalized.

Smartphone-based applications. There are more and more devices and applications available that can work with your smartphone or home computer. Some are devices that simply measure your heart rate and can give an indication of an abnormal rhythm. Other devices are more sophisticated and can actually provide a *rhythm strip* similar to what we can obtain with Holter monitors. The rhythm strip is a short two- to ten-second recording of your heart rhythm that looks like a single lead on an ECG. It can often be used to diagnose an arrhythmia. An example of a smartphone-based device is the AliveCor Kardia Mobile ECG app (AliveCor, Inc., San Francisco, CA), and another option that can actually be used as a stand-alone device to record a short segment of your heart rhythm is the HeartCheck PEN handheld ECG (CardioComm Solutions, Inc., North York, ON, Canada).

Tilt-table test. Your doctor may order a tilt-table test to look for causes of fainting (syncope). In this test, you lie on a table with your legs straight. The table is then elevated at an angle so that your head is higher than your feet. You are kept in this position for several minutes to assess for the development of symptoms such as fainting or palpitations. Your response to the tilt-table test may enable your doctor to tailor therapy to treat your symptoms. Medications such as beta-blockers, midodrine, or fludrocortisone may be prescribed in response to an abnormal tilt-table test.

Implantable loop recorders. Implantable loop recorders offer your doctor a means to assess for heart-rhythm abnormalities with conditions that occur infrequently and *in patients who experience fainting or loss of consciousness.* Many arrhythmias only occur once a month or only a few times a year. Sometimes, it is very difficult to document an arrhythmia or assess for the cause of syncope (fainting) if we are using Holter monitors (which can record your heart rhythm for twenty-four to forty-eight hours) or even the two- to four-week outpatient telemetry monitors described previously. These devices continuously record several minutes of your heart rhythm (this is called a *loop recording*); when the device detects a possible heart-rhythm abnormality or the patient "activates" the device, this loop of the heart-rhythm recording is saved to the device's memory chip. The recordings are then downloaded from the device at your doctor's office or transmitted to your doctor's office from your home (if this feature is included in your device). Figure 5 in chapter 2 shows a portion of a heart rhythm (the top tracing) that can typically be recorded by these devices.

There are several types of implantable loop recorders, and examples are shown in figure 6. These devices are typically implanted under the skin of the left chest overlying your heart. Clearly, the closer your heart is to the device, the better are the recordings of the electrical signals coming from your heart. Once the loop recorder is implanted, it is capable of continuously monitoring your heart rhythm for several years (I usually estimate a device longevity of two to four years). The device has a built-in battery as well as the circuitry necessary to run the device and make heart-rhythm recordings. The implanting physician (or your cardiologist) generally programs the device to automatically record heart rates less than 40 beats per minute (bpm) or above 150 bpm; talk to your doctor because these settings may be customized for a particular patient's needs. Furthermore, most of these devices permit patients to "activate" the device if they are experiencing worrisome symptoms.

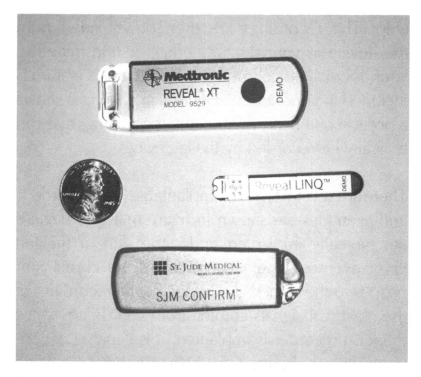

Figure 6. Implantable Loop Recorders. These small devices are implanted under the skin below the collarbone in the left chest region. They can record heart rhythms to allow the patient and care provider to determine if any symptoms are caused by abnormally fast or slow heart rhythms. They monitor heart rhythm continuously, twenty-four hours a day, and have a longevity of two to four years. They are used only to assess the rhythm and do not function as pacemakers or deliver any therapy.

When you feel a symptom that may be caused by an abnormal heart rhythm, you press a button on a device (about the size of a pager) you can carry in your pocket or purse. Pressing the activation button triggers the device to store a recording of your heart rhythm (during your symptoms), which can then be examined by your care provider. These electrical recordings of your heart rhythm can document (for your doctor's review) a normal heart rhythm abruptly converting to a fast (or slow) arrhythmia that may be contributing to your symptoms. Conversely, the recordings may also demonstrate that your symptoms are not associated with any abnormal arrhythmia.

An emerging use of implantable loop recorders is for patients who experience strokes with no obvious cause (called cryptogenic stroke). Strokes are "brain attacks" and may also be called a transient ischemic attack (TIA) or cerebrovascular accident (CVA). One in ten patients may have a stroke caused by atrial fibrillation. One-third of patients with atrial fibrillation may not have any symptoms suggesting arrhythmia other than a stroke. A loop recorder may be recommended to detect atrial fibrillation in a patient with risk factors for atrial fibrillation who have had a stroke.

Summary. You can see that your doctor has many options for assessing heart-rhythm abnormalities. Every patient is different, and the evaluation for arrhythmia has to be tailored to each patient, with careful attention to the patient's symptoms. For a patient who experiences daily arrhythmia symptoms, the best way to detect an arrhythmia may be a twenty-four-hour Holter monitor, whereas a patient who faints once or twice per year may be best evaluated with the use of an implantable loop recorder. It is generally preferable to start with noninvasive methods (e.g., twenty-four-hour Holter and MCOT) prior to considering an implantable loop recorder. It is important to discuss these options with your care providers.

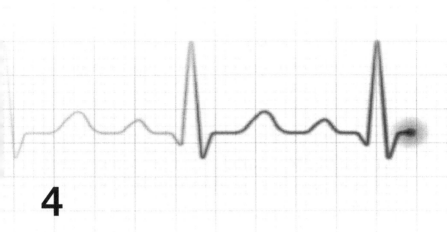

4

Work-up and Evaluation of Heart-Rhythm Disorders (Meeting the Heart-Rhythm Physician)

Introduction. The first important element of the evaluation for heart-rhythm disorders is the type of care provider who will be performing the evaluation. Care providers have varying years of training built upon a foundation of patient evaluation that permits a thorough, yet concise, summary of a patient and his or her symptoms, medical history, and differential diagnosis. The differential diagnosis consists of the possible diagnoses (in order of likelihood) that can explain the patient's constellation of symptoms. There is a wide variety of providers—with a wide variety of training backgrounds—who can evaluate you for a heart-rhythm disorder, such as the following:

- *Physician assistants* have about three years of health-care experience and a bachelor's degree before they obtain their physician assistant certification by attending school for an additional two years.
- *Nurse practitioners* are registered nurses who have completed a master's or doctoral degree program and have advanced clinical training beyond their initial professional registered nurse preparation.
- A *family practice doctor* has completed four years of undergraduate college, four years of medical school, and three years of a family practice residency. These professionals usually see both children and adults.
- An *internal medicine doctor* (also called *internist*) has completed four years of undergraduate college, four years of medical school, and three years of an internal medicine residency. These professionals usually see only adults.
- A *cardiologist* is an internal medicine doctor whose training involves four years of undergraduate college, four years of medical school, three years of internal medicine

residency, and three years of cardiology fellowship. Many cardiologists are board certified in internal medicine and cardiology.

- An *electrophysiologist* is a subspecialized cardiologist who performs heart-rhythm evaluations and procedures to implant electrophysiology (EP) devices—such as pacemakers and defibrillators. Typical training involves the same training as that for a cardiologist, plus an additional two years of EP (heart rhythm) fellowship. During this EP fellowship, an electrophysiologist focuses exclusively on pacemaker and defibrillator implantation as well as the long-term care of these devices. In addition, an electrophysiologist is trained in all aspects of heart-rhythm evaluation and care, including EP studies and heart ablations to cure various arrhythmias. Many electrophysiologists are board certified in internal medicine, cardiology, and clinical cardiac electrophysiology.

History of present illness (HPI). The most important element of evaluating a patient is an open discussion to determine the present illness. It is estimated that over 80 percent of patients can be diagnosed just by obtaining an accurate history from the patient (Hampton et al. 1975). One of the most important aspects of the evaluation of a patient with symptoms suggestive of arrhythmia is whether or not the patient is at risk for or has been appropriately treated for significant underlying heart disease, such as obstructive coronary-artery disease. Symptoms such as loss of consciousness (syncope), dizziness, shortness of breath, chest pain, palpitations, or exertional fatigue can all be related to heart-rhythm disorders with underlying structural heart disease.

Typical Patient HPI: The patient is a seventy-two-year-old white female who has had eleven episodes of sudden loss of consciousness over the past four years. She has had seizure activity witnessed by others, and under the care of her primary-care physician, neurologist, and general cardiologist, she has been started on an anti-seizure medicine. She continues to experience episodes of syncope. Each episode involves a short period of dizziness and blacking out. This is followed by a loss of consciousness. More often than not, these episodes are abrupt in their onset, occur without much warning, and have resulted in injury at times. They can occur while the patient is seated or standing. They do not appear to be related to meals, dehydration,

> *emotional stress, or any other obvious cause. There are no related symptoms, such as chest pain, shortness of breath, or rapid heartbeat.*

Common elements of the HPI. We can describe the HPI using seven categories to encompass all elements of the history. COLDER-AS is a mnemonic used to ensure that all the right questions are asked when evaluating a patient and stands for **C**haracter, **O**nset, **L**ocation, **D**uration, **E**xacerbating factors, **R**elieving factors, and **A**ssociated **S**ymptoms (see table 2).

Character concerns the subjective elements of the symptom or problem. Each of the remaining elements is then used to describe the particular issue for a complete description. The HPI can be gathered by anyone familiar with patient care. Physician extenders—such as nurse practitioners, physician assistants, nurses, or medical assistants—may gather this background information. It is not so much how the information is obtained; rather, what is important is that *all* the information is obtained.

Table 2. Major Elements in the History of Present Illness

Character	The characteristics of the symptoms (e.g., pressure, burning, aching)
Onset	Circumstances/timing of symptoms
Location	Where is the pain felt, and is it felt in any other locations?
Duration	How long have the symptoms been present, and how long do they last?
Exacerbating factors	What has the patient done to aggravate the symptom (walking, sitting, standing, eating, drinking, etc.)?
Relieving factors	What has the patient done to relieve the symptom (deep breathing, cold water, nitroglycerin, belching, aspirin, etc.)?
Associated Symptoms	What are the symptoms that the patient notices to occur at same time as the main issue? (Examples include shortness of breath, heart racing, sweating, nausea, vomiting, etc.)

Past medical and surgical history (PMH). The past medical and surgical history helps to "risk stratify" patients. Elements of a patient history—including prior heart attacks (myocardial infarction [MI]), congestive heart failure (CHF), or arrhythmias such as ventricular tachycardia/fibrillation and atrial fibrillation—suggest underlying heart disease and possibly increased risk of arrhythmia. In addition, there are other, noncardiac medical problems that can hint at risk factors for arrhythmias. Peripheral vascular disease (blockages in arteries such as the carotids in the neck or arteries in the legs) can also indicate that heart disease is present. Not only can coronary arteries get plaques (or fatty blockages), but the heart's conduction and muscle system can also be diseased by a buildup of calcification and/or fibrous scar tissue. Finally, there are a host of medical conditions that can increase the risk of arrhythmia, such as the following:

- *Thyroid*: Both an underactive (hypothyroidism) and an overactive (hyperthyroidism) thyroid can lead to heart-rhythm abnormalities. Usually, a blood lab test that evaluates the level of thyroid-stimulating hormone (TSH) is ordered; an abnormally high or low TSH can be treated and possibly eliminate heart-rhythm problems.
- *Hypertension*: Elevated blood pressure can lead to arrhythmias (commonly, atrial fibrillation), and normalizing blood pressure may help decrease heart-rhythm abnormalities.
- *Coronary-artery disease*: Rarely, blockages in the coronary arteries can lead to arrhythmias,

and these blockages are usually associated with chest pain, shortness of breath, or other symptoms that occur with physical exertion.

- *Infections*: Any infection can lead to arrhythmias. Treating the underlying infection often relieves the arrhythmia.
- *Myocarditis/pericarditis*: Inflammation or infection of the heart muscle (myocarditis) or the heart's outer lining (pericarditis) may cause arrhythmias.
- *Pulmonary conditions*: Lung disease can place excess strain on your heart, and conditions such as pneumonia or blood clots (pulmonary embolism) may lead to arrhythmias.
- *Alcohol*: Alcohol is a direct toxin to your heart and can lead to arrhythmias. In some cases, excess alcohol intake on special occasions (we call this "holiday heart") can lead to transient arrhythmias. Chronic excessive use of alcohol can lead to heart failure and long-term issues with arrhythmias.
- *Drugs*: Use of any illicit substance, such as cocaine, heroin, and marijuana, can lead to arrhythmias. In addition, any toxic ingestion or overdose could lead to arrhythmias.

Social history. The "social" history is used to obtain details of a person's life that are not purely medical.

Personal habits such as the use of tobacco (causing vascular disease), alcohol, and illicit drugs—which are toxic to the heart muscle and cause heart-rhythm abnormalities—raise the suspicion of serious heart problems. Additionally, personal stresses—such as deaths in the family, marital issues, or the loss of a job—can increase stress. *Many heart-rhythm abnormalities are exacerbated by increased stress, decreased sleep, and use of caffeine, alcohol, or nicotine. Conversely, regular exercise, a healthy diet, good sleep habits, smoking cessation, and weight loss can decrease heart-rhythm abnormalities.*

Family history. The saying "an apple does not fall far from the tree" is used to emphasize the importance of family history. We are trained to specifically ask for family histories of heart disease and the ages at which it occurred. The relative must be a blood relative (not an in-law), and we are mainly concerned with *first-degree relatives*, namely, mother, father, sister, and brother. Common heart problems that can be transmitted across generations include coronary-artery disease, heart attacks, atrial fibrillation, and sudden cardiac death.

Sudden cardiac death refers to an unexpected (and sometimes at a very young age) death that was likely related to the heart. Additional family histories that may suggest sudden cardiac death include "unexplained" seizure disorders and drownings in relatives who knew how to swim. During sudden cardiac death, the heart muscle stops pumping, causing the brain to experience a lack of oxygen and possible seizure. Family members who have experienced sudden cardiac death and miraculously recover in seconds may be misdiagnosed with seizure disorders. In addition, some conditions that can cause sudden cardiac death are triggered by vigorous exertion (e.g., long-QT syndrome); if a person with such a condition was swimming when sudden cardiac death occurred, the death may be mistakenly called a drowning.

Physical exam (including vital signs). Vital signs include heart rate (heartbeats per minute), blood pressure, respiratory rate (breaths per minute), and pulse oximetry (pulse ox), which measures the oxygen content of blood.

Heart rate. A normal range for the resting heart rate is sixty to one hundred beats per minute (bpm). *Bradycardia* refers to a heart rate of less than 60 bpm, but very physically fit people can have normally slow resting heart rates of less than 60 bpm. *Tachycardia* refers to a heart rate of more than 100 bpm. Generally, your heart rate accelerates to between 100 and 120 bpm during a brisk walk or when climbing steps (called *sinus tachycardia*), and this is a normal response to exercise. An abnormally slow response to exercise—an inability to get the heart rate above 100 bpm, with associated chest pain or shortness of breath—can indicate sinus-node dysfunction and is called *chronotropic incompetence*. Abnormally fast heart rates can indicate abnormal heart rhythms that need medical treatment. The following box describes a very common arrhythmia that can result in significant heart-rate variation.

What is atrial fibrillation? Atrial fibrillation (AF) is the most common arrhythmia seen in a typical electrophysiology practice and often presents with an abnormal or irregular heart rate. Almost 5 percent (five out of one hundred) of patients older than sixty years of age have AF, and the percentage increases almost 0.5 percent per year so that by eighty years of age, up to 15 percent of people may have AF. Atrial fibrillation refers to the top chambers of the heart (the right and left atria) fibrillating (or beating rapidly) at 300 to 400 bpm. This rapid beating is transmitted to the lower pumping chambers of the heart (ventricles) and causes most of the symptoms *attributed to AF, such as palpitations, heart racing, chest pain, and shortness of breath. The most concerning aspect of AF—aside from the aforementioned symptoms—is the risk of stroke (blood clots sent to the brain). Atrial fibrillation causes the atria to stop contracting and just quiver. This loss of pumping can lead to blood-clot formation in an atrium. The diagnosis of AF (or atrial flutter, a closely related heart-rhythm disorder) should lead you to a discussion with your doctor about anticoagulation to prevent the development of strokes.*

Blood pressure. The ideal blood pressure in most patients is 120 over 80. The top number is called the *systolic* blood pressure, and the bottom number is called the *diastolic* blood pressure. When a patient has elevated blood pressure, changes in diet and increased exercise can often normalize blood pressure. Sometimes, changes in diet and exercise are not enough, and most doctors treat blood pressures above 140 over 90 with medication. Recent research suggests that extremely elderly patients (age greater than eighty years) may have a higher target blood pressure.

Respiratory rate. The respiratory rate refers to how often a person breathes in one minute. The normal rate is approximately eight to fourteen breaths per minute. Shortness of breath (or difficulty breathing) is often associated with an increased respiratory rate.

Pulse oximetry. Pulse oximetry is used to determine the oxygen saturation in the blood. Normal oxygen saturation is greater than 95 percent. Heart patients can have abnormal (low) pulse-oximetry readings due to the presence of heart failure (or chronic obstructive pulmonary disease [COPD]).

Weight. Weight is important to obtain because patients who have heart failure will often gain weight. Close monitoring of weight can allow a patient to alert his or her doctor of an impending heart-failure exacerbation. Generally, rapid weight gain (or loss) of more than two to three pounds in several days corresponds to fluid weight. In addition, abnormally high or low body weights may place patients at higher risk of heart-rhythm abnormalities.

Pertinent studies. There are many tests that your care provider may want to obtain to evaluate your symptoms. A *chest radiograph,* or chest x-ray, is obtained to ensure that the lungs and heart are in suitable condition, with no obvious abnormalities. The *electrocardiogram* (EKG) is obtained to evaluate for any heart-rhythm disorders or electrical-system blockages. See figure 7 for examples of normal and abnormal EKGs. An echocardiogram (*echo* for short) is used to assess for any decline in heart-pumping function (ejection fraction [EF]) as well as to assess for heart-chamber sizes and any valve disease. *Stress tests* may be performed prior to an echocardiogram to assess symptoms that may indicate coronary-artery blockages. Reasons for stress tests include the following: (1) to see if symptoms such as chest pain or shortness of breath are due to underlying coronary-artery blockages or (2) to assess for possible side effects of antiarrhythmic medications. Finally, *baseline blood laboratory tests*—such as kidney function, blood counts, and blood-coagulation studies—are performed to make sure there are no other medical conditions contributing to heart-rhythm disorders.

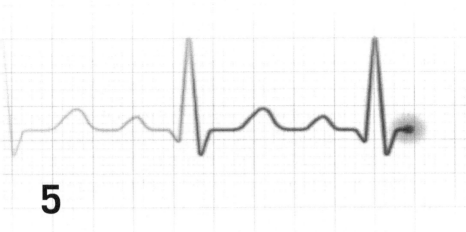

5

What Are the Common Supraventricular (Top-Chamber) Tachycardias?

Introduction. The incidence of arrhythmias varies depending on region and type of practice. An inner-city heart-rhythm doctor may see different arrhythmias than a more rural cardiologist. Figure 4 in chapter 2 shows the frequency and types of arrhythmias seen in all patients (figure 4A) and those arrhythmias encountered when performing electrophysiology (EP) studies and ablations during my first two years of practice when I started a new heart-rhythm program in a rural community in 2008 (figure 4B; Chow et al. 2012; Williams et al. 201). The most common arrhythmia I encountered in the EP laboratory was atrioventricular nodal reentrant tachycardia (AVNRT). It must be noted that the most common arrhythmia I see in my overall practice is atrial fibrillation; however, I try to manage atrial fibrillation medically before considering an ablation. This explains the relatively low rate of atrial fibrillation in my patients who undergo an ablation. You can also see from figure 4B that ventricular tachycardia (discussed in chapter 7) is much less common. Any of these arrhythmias can be triggered by increased stress, decreased sleep, and use of caffeine, alcohol, illicit drugs, or nicotine.

Please keep in mind that the incidence rates of heart-rhythm abnormalities shown in figure 4B represent arrhythmias in very symptomatic patients who were brought to the EP laboratory in an attempt to cure the arrhythmias. There are many arrhythmias that may not be routinely "cured," such as atrial fibrillation and ventricular tachycardia. This chapter discusses each of the most common arrhythmias and their treatment options.

Premature atrial contractions. Premature atrial contractions (PACs) may also be called atrial premature contractions (APCs) or atrial premature depolarizations (APDs). These are extra signals from the top chambers (atria) that can trigger an extra heartbeat that interrupts the regular rhythm. These have been found to occur in 97 percent of healthy patients older than sixty-five years of age within a twenty-four-hour period (Chow et al. 2012). They are generally harmless, although they may cause symptoms if they occur frequently.

AV-node reentrant tachycardia. AVNRT is a supra-ventricular tachycardia (SVT) that can be seen as short, asymptomatic bursts in up to 50 percent of healthy patients over the age of sixty-five. I have seen this arrhythmia in over 30 percent of patients who underwent an EP study and ablation. Most people have a single electrical channel (also called pathway) in the AV node that transmits electrical impulses from the atria to the ventricles. However, 10 to 35 percent of people may have what is called *dual AV-node physiology*. Most people with dual AV-node physiology are not even aware that they have this condition, but a small percentage of patients can develop AVNRT as a result of these dual pathways. Normal day-to-day heart rhythms use the faster of the two pathways. Occasionally, a normal electrical impulse traverses from the atria to the ventricles using the *slower pathway* and then immediately sends an electrical signal back up to the atria from the ventricles via the *faster pathway*. If this continues heartbeat after heartbeat, the patient will experience a fast arrhythmia and may develop symptoms such as palpitations. There are several different types of AVNRT, but all types can be treated by performing an ablation of the slow AV-node pathway, leaving the fast AV-node pathway intact.

AV reentrant tachycardia. AV reentrant tachycardia is an SVT caused by an accessory pathway (outside the AV node) that causes an abnormal, extra connection between the top (atria) and bottom (ventricles). This tends to be discovered in childhood or as a young adult but can be found in older patients as well. Interestingly, I have had several older patients who experienced symptoms of palpitations for decades (with some including various outpatient monitors and multiple emergency room visits) but were never able to demonstrate the arrhythmia to their care providers. I tell my patients, "Sometimes the car doesn't make that noise when you bring it to the mechanic!" *Wolff-Parkinson-White* (WPW) syndrome is a rare type of arrhythmia in which a patient has AV reentrant tachycardia causing palpitations and a special type of electrocardiogram (ECG) abnormality called preexcitation. This is often diagnosed in childhood but may be found later in life. Appendix 1 helps explain the differenc between AVNRT and AVRT.

Common Clinical Scenario 1

A fifty-two-year-old woman presented for evaluation after over thirty years of palpitations. She reported episodes of the sudden onset of a fast and regular heart racing. The episodes seemed to have no obvious triggering or relieving factors and usually resolved on their own in five to ten minutes. She occasionally had success in terminating the symptoms with vagal maneuvers. (discussed in chapter 8). Vagal maneuvers include things like bearing down as if you were having a bowel movement, coughing vigorously, and placing your face in a bowl of ice water. Multiple outpatient and emergency room (ER) visits over the years as well as ECGs and Holter monitoring had not uncovered any arrhythmias because the episodes only occurred every few months. Trials with beta-blockers and calcium-channel blockers were not effective in relieving her symptoms. I advised her to immediately come to the office for any recurrent symptoms, and she subsequently presented to the office with an SVT of 220 beats per minute (bpm; normal heart rate is less than 100 bpm). She ultimately decided to have an EP study, and we successfully ablated AV-node reentrant tachycardia and an accessory pathway causing AV reentrant tachycardia as well. It is not common to have two types of arrhythmias, but she became symptom-free after the ablation.

Atrial tachycardia. Atrial tachycardia is an SVT caused by an abnormal focus (or cluster) of cells in the top chamber of the heart (atria) that fires irregularly and randomly. AT is further explained in Appendix 2.

Atrial flutter. This SVT is the "first cousin" of atrial fibrillation and may also lead to an increased risk of stroke (discussed in chapter 6). It can be very difficult to control medically and may require electrical cardioversion or an ablation (which can possibly cure atrial flutter). Appendix 3 helps explain the difference between atrial flutter and atrial fibrillation.

<u>Common Clinical Scenario 2</u>

A seventy-two-year-old man presented for evaluation of palpitations from typical atrial flutter. He was seen by a general cardiologist and was found to have a new diagnosis of atrial flutter about six months prior. The patient was placed on warfarin and metoprolol and underwent a cardioversion with a preceding transesophageal echo (which showed no evidence of a blood clot in his heart). He was successfully cardioverted back into his normal sinus rhythm at that time, but about one month before the current visit, he had a recurrence of palpitations and was found to have returned to atrial flutter. He underwent an EP study and successful ablation for typical atrial flutter while continuing his warfarin uninterrupted.

Atrial fibrillation. Atrial fibrillation is the most common arrhythmia encountered in cardiology practice. It is caused by the abnormally fast beating (fibrillation) of the top chambers of the heart (atria). This fibrillation triggers the bottom chambers of the heart (ventricles) to beat very fast, causing symptoms. The next chapter discusses atrial fibrillation and its treatment, but anti-coagulation to decrease the risk of stroke followed by medications to control heart rate are the usual first steps in management.

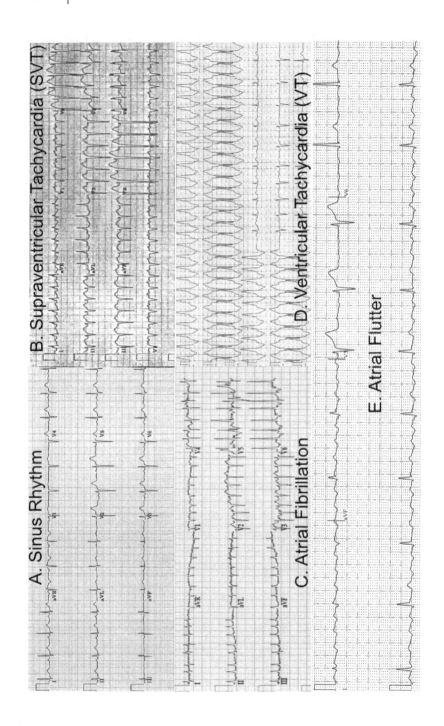

A. Sinus Rhythm

B. Supraventricular Tachycardia (SVT)

C. Atrial Fibrillation

D. Ventricular Tachycardia (VT)

E. Atrial Flutter

Figure 7. Electrocardiograms of Common Arrhythmias. Panel A, shows normal sinus rhythm, which is the heart's baseline rhythm; the tall, narrow spikes are the QRS complexes. Panel B shows what a supraventricular tachycardia (in this case, atrioventricular nodal reentrant tachycardia) looks like; notice how narrow the QRS complex is. Panel C shows atrial fibrillation with the very irregular-appearing QRS complexes. Panel D shows ventricular tachycardia; note the very wide QRS complexes, especially when compared to the narrow QRS complexes after the VT stops. The main difference between SVT and VT is the wide QRS complexes, but some SVTs may have wide QRS complexes (this is called *aberrancy*). Panel E shows atrial flutter, which has a "sawtooth" appearance of the baseline between QRS complexes. Atrial flutter is treated using the same techniques and medicines as those for atrial fibrillation.

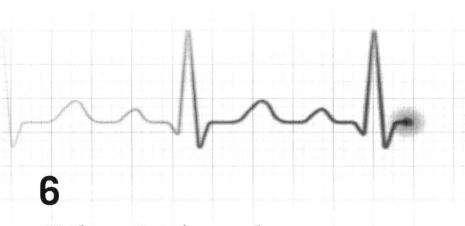

6
What Is Atrial Fibrillation?

Introduction. Atrial fibrillation is the most common clinical arrhythmia encountered in cardiac electrophysiology, and it is a problem of the top chambers in your heart—that is, the atria. Approximately 5 percent of people over sixty years of age have atrial fibrillation! If you have atrial fibrillation, your most significant risk is for stroke, and the first step in treatment is deciding what type of anticoagulation is appropriate for your situation. Aspirin alone may be adequate, but you may require warfarin or one of the newer oral anticoagulants that can be used in place of warfarin (e.g., Coumadin). There are "triggers" for atrial fibrillation that are primarily located in the pulmonary veins connected to the left atrium;

these electrical "triggers" are called pulmonary vein potentials. There are many complex mechanisms that underlie how the electrical properties of pulmonary veins may cause atrial fibrillation. We are still learning about the science of how the pulmonary veins are linked to atrial fibrillation; the advancement of this science may result in the development of better treatments and perhaps a cure for atrial fibrillation. The next issue is to determine how to manage the heart-rhythm abnormality itself.

A *rhythm-control* strategy is in place when you are given *antiarrhythmics* (medications that help maintain a normal rhythm) to prevent atrial fibrillation from happening; this strategy is ideal for patients with severe symptoms. Antiarrhythmics include flecainide, propafenone, amiodarone, sotalol, dofetilide, and dronedarone.

A *rate-control* strategy allows the presence of atrial fibrillation but prevents fast heart rates with medications to slow your heart rate; this is a good option for patients who do not feel their atrial fibrillation (*three out of ten patients with atrial fibrillation may not have symptoms*). Medications to help slow your heart while you are in atrial fibrillation include beta-blockers (e.g., metoprolol, atenolol, and carvedilol), calcium-channel blockers (e.g., diltiazem and verapamil), and digoxin.

The most important thing to realize is that atrial fibrillation will not be completely treated (or understood) in a single visit. Be patient with your care provider. A medicine that works for one patient may not work for another.

Normal electrical activation versus atrial fibrillation. The normal electrical activation of the heart is described in chapter 1 (see figure 3). The *P wave* corresponds to the electrical activation of the right and left atria. The P wave then triggers the bottom chambers (the ventricles) to beat and pump blood to the rest of the body. Each P wave corresponds to one heartbeat during normal electrical activation. During atrial fibrillation, the atria beat very fast and irregularly (called fibrillation). Thus, instead of one P wave triggering the bottom chambers approximately once per second, the bottom chambers receive five or six signals per second! This atrial fibrillation can then cause your bottom chambers to beat at approximately 100 to 200 beats per minute (bpm). Figure 7 in chapter 5 shows a normal sinus rhythm (panel A) versus the fast and irregular rhythm when atrial fibrillation is present (panel C).

Signs and symptoms. When your heart beats irregularly and faster than 100 bpm, you can have symptoms such as chest pain, shortness of breath, palpitations, dizziness, and fatigue. It must be noted that atrial fibrillation can cause symptoms even if your heart rate is less than 100 bpm. Atrial fibrillation usually causes an irregular heartbeat; however, one-third of patients may not have any symptoms.

Causes of atrial fibrillation. When I encounter a patient with atrial fibrillation, I look for a host of other possible causes of atrial fibrillation in addition to evaluating a patient for increased stress, decreased sleep, and use of caffeine, alcohol, and nicotine. A common mnemonic to help remember all the causes of atrial fibrillation is THIMPAD:

- **T**hyroid: An overactive thyroid can trigger atrial fibrillation, and your doctor will generally screen for thyroid issues by checking your levels of thyroid-stimulating hormone (TSH).
- **H**ypertension: High blood pressure can put a strain on your heart (specifically, the atria) and lead to atrial fibrillation. Oftentimes, patients are admitted to the hospital for atrial fibrillation with rapid heart rates, and simply

controlling the blood pressure can terminate the atrial fibrillation.

- Ischemia/Infection: Ischemia refers to active coronary-artery disease (e.g., blockages in your coronary arteries) that may rarely lead to atrial fibrillation. Also, any infection could increase your body's inflammatory state and trigger atrial fibrillation.
- Myocarditis: Inflammation of your heart muscle during or after a viral illness could lead to atrial fibrillation.
- Pulmonary issues: Any strain on your lungs (such as pneumonia, chronic obstructive pulmonary disease, or obstructive sleep apnea) could lead to atrial fibrillation.
- Alcohol: Alcohol is a direct toxin to your heart and can lead to atrial fibrillation and even heart failure.
- Drugs: Use of illicit drugs, such as marijuana, cocaine, or methamphetamines, can lead to atrial fibrillation.

Congestive heart failure (CHF) can be a cause of atrial fibrillation; conversely, atrial fibrillation can cause heart failure. As discussed earlier, patients with heart failure have increased strain placed on the heart and this can lead to atrial fibrillation. Less commonly, atrial fibrillation can lead to sustained periods of fast heart rates that can cause heart failure.

Obesity is such an important risk factor for atrial fibrillation that I have to talk about it separately from other issues. Obesity is defined as a body mass index (BMI) greater than 30 kg/m². BMI is a tool that takes height into account to "standardize" weight assessment. Morbid obesity is defined as a BMI greater than 40 kg/m². Obesity has a multitude of ill effects on the body: increased blood pressure, increased inflammatory "milieu" of the body, increased levels of "bad" cholesterol, and increased risk of diabetes. These can then increase a person's risk of coronary and peripheral vascular disease, obstructive sleep apnea, and hypertensive heart disease. Obstructive sleep apnea (OSA) is a particularly potent trigger for atrial fibrillation. OSA decreases the amount of oxygen in the blood, increases inflammation, and increases pressures inside your heart. These can all, in turn, increase the risk for atrial fibrillation. Weight loss has been shown to decrease the frequency of atrial fibrillation episodes (secondary prevention) *and* prevent the first occurrence of atrial fibrillation (primary prevention). See table 3 for an easy screening tool to see if you are at risk for OSA.

Table 3. STOP-BANG Assessment to Screen for Obstructive Sleep Apnea

STOP	
Do you **S**nore loudly?	Yes No
Do you often feel **T**ired, sleepy, or fatigued during the daytime?	Yes No
Has anyone **O**bserved you stop breathing during sleep?	Yes No
Do you have or are you being treated for high blood **P**ressure?	Yes No
BANG	
BMI more than 35 kg/m^2?	Yes No
AGE greater than fifty years?	Yes No
NECK circumference > 16 in.?	Yes No
GENDER male?	Yes No
TOTAL SCORE	

Scoring key: High risk of obstructive sleep apnea: Yes 5–8

Intermediate risk of obstructive sleep apnea: Yes 3–4

Low risk of obstructive sleep apnea: Yes 0–2

You can see from the exhaustive list of possible causes why I consider atrial fibrillation a "symptom" of other disease. I try to find reversible causes of atrial fibrillation prior to considering medications such as antiarrhythmics. Some patients are described as having "lone" atrial fibrillation. Lone atrial fibrillation means that we can't find any obvious trigger or cause for atrial fibrillation, and it may be more common in younger patients with atrial fibrillation.

People often ask me, "What causes atrial fibrillation?" You can see how this can be a difficult question to answer in a single office visit. I often tell patients that the person who can answer that question (or come up with the "cure") will get a Nobel Prize! There are many diseases a doctor needs to check for when you have atrial fibrillation, but the doctor may not find a clear cause for your atrial fibrillation. We do understand that there are "triggers" for atrial fibrillation that are primarily located in the pulmonary veins connected to the left atrium. Ablation can be used to prevent these triggers from starting atrial fibrillation. The goal of electrically isolating (preventing electrical communication between your left atrium and) your pulmonary veins by performing an ablation is to help decrease the burden of atrial fibrillation. The electrical triggers for atrial fibrillation can be located in many other places in your right and left atrium which may help explain why there is no "cure" for atrial fibrillation by ablation at this time.

Understanding your risk of stroke. Your risk of stroke varies depending on the risk factors you may have. Risk-stratification systems have been developed to help care providers determine which patients are at the highest risk of stroke and may need more than just aspirin as an anticoagulant (aka blood thinner). Table 4 provides an example of a risk-scoring system called the CHA2DS2-VASc.

Table 4. CHA2DS2-VASc Score to Assess Risk of Stroke

Risk	Score
Congestive Heart Failure	1
Hypertension	1
Age ≥ 75 or older	2
Diabetes	1
Stroke (TIA)	2
Vascular Disease*	1
Age 65–74 Years	1
Sex Female	1

*Prior myocardial infarction, peripheral artery disease, aortic plaque. TIA=transient ischemic attack.

Generally, a CHA2DS2-VASc score of 1 or more implies that aspirin alone may not be adequate. If your risk factors merit more than aspirin alone, your doctor will likely discuss several options for anticoagulation.

Warfarin (Coumadin) is a once-daily pill that requires regular blood laboratory tests to monitor the lab value called the International Normalized Ratio (INR) to help determine how much warfarin you should take on a daily basis. A normal INR value is 1, and we generally try to keep patients at an INR value between 2 and 3. Every patient is different, and patients may require very different daily doses of warfarin. Furthermore, warfarin may interact with a host of different medications, and any change in medication may necessitate a change in warfarin dosing. Antibiotics and medications such as amiodarone can cause dramatic changes in INR values.

Target specific oral anticoagulants (TSOACs) are a new class of medications that are taken once or twice daily and do not require routine blood laboratory tests. These medications include dabigatran (Pradaxa), apixaban (Eliquis), and rivaroxaban (Xarelto); more of these types of medications are becoming available each year. Each of these medications requires your doctor to discuss the pros and cons of stroke prevention weighed against the risk of bleeding. Any medication (including aspirin) that thins your blood to prevent blood clotting can increase your risk of bleeding.

It is important to discuss your risks of stroke and anti-coagulation options with your care provider!

Is there a difference between atrial fibrillation and ventricular fibrillation? Atrial fibrillation and ventricular fibrillation are *very* different. *Ventricular tachycardia* refers to a very fast beating of the bottom chambers of the heart (the ventricles) and can cause low blood pressure, loss of consciousness, and even death if not treated. *Ventricular fibrillation* refers to an even faster beating of the bottom chambers of the heart (ventricles) and is often fatal. During *sudden cardiac death*, when the heart goes into ventricular fibrillation, the bottom chambers just quiver, and no blood is pumped. This leads to a loss of blood pressure, followed by loss of consciousness (called *syncope* or fainting) and then, if not stopped quickly, death. It may seem confusing, but it is possible to survive sudden cardiac death. A person can faint because of sudden cardiac death (e.g., ventricular fibrillation) and be revived quickly, depending on the underlying medical condition and availability of emergency personnel.

Figure 5 in chapter 2 shows the electrocardiogram of a patient who had an episode of ventricular fibrillation while hospitalized. This patient quickly underwent electrical *cardioversion* and had a defibrillator placed to stop further episodes of ventricular fibrillation. Cardioversion is a procedure using electricity (as in this case) or medicines to convert an abnormally fast heart rhythm to a normal rhythm.

Is there a cure for atrial fibrillation? Unfortunately, there is no "cure" for atrial fibrillation. We can use medicines and even ablation to help decrease your symptom burden from atrial fibrillation. Some patients can go several years without atrial fibrillation symptoms from medicines and/or ablation, but there is no cure for the condition. The appropriate course of action is to try antiarrhythmic medications before considering an invasive treatment such as ablation; ablations for atrial fibrillation (as opposed to other types of supraventricular tachycardia [SVT], including atrial flutter) can entail significant risk. If a particular antiarrhythmic does not work for a patient, I usually try a different one. Not all patients respond to medications the same, and an antiarrhythmic that worked for one patient may not work for another patient. If the atrial fibrillation is not causing symptoms such as chest pain, shortness of breath, or palpitations, then the most important strategy is decreasing the risk of stroke with anticoagulation and ensuring that heart rates are adequately controlled.

Common Clinical Scenario 3

A seventy-four-year-old woman with no significant past medical history was found to have atrial fibrillation causing severe symptoms of palpitations and shortness of breath, as confirmed with a twenty-four-hour Holter monitor. She had a CHA2DS2-VASc score of 2 and was tolerating treatment with dabigatran (Pradaxa) without obvious bleeding. She initially presented with symptomatic paroxysmal atrial fibrillation and was placed on anticoagulation as well as metoprolol and flecainide. Several months later, she was readmitted to the hospital with highly symptomatic atrial fibrillation (lasting eight to twenty-four hours) breaking through the flecainide. Her flecainide was changed to Tikosyn (dofetilide), and she required a cardioversion to return to her normal sinus rhythm. At that time, we talked about considering ablation versus continued attempts with antiarrhythmic medications; she opted for continued attempts at medical management. She had further episodes of atrial fibrillation and required a change from dofetilide to sotalol, only to present several weeks later with highly symptomatic atrial fibrillation lasting eight to twenty-four hours. After trying multiple antiarrhythmics, the patient ultimately decided to proceed with an atrial fibrillation ablation, which was performed without any major complications. After the procedure, she still experienced periods of atrial fibrillation, but they were less frequent and occurred with less severe symptoms, and she was happy with this level of improvement because the symptoms no longer significantly disrupted her life.

What is atrial flutter? Atrial flutter is like a "first cousin" to atrial fibrillation. Panel E of Figure 7 in chapter 5 shows what atrial flutter looks like on an electrocardiogram (ECG or EKG). First and foremost, *we treat the risks of stroke from atrial flutter the same way as in atrial fibrillation.* In fact, up to 60 to 70 percent of patients with atrial flutter have likely had atrial fibrillation within the past year. Typical (located in the right atrium) atrial flutter can be easily cured (>95 percent cure rate) with catheter ablation, whereas nontypical (located in the left atrium) atrial flutter is not as easily cured. Sometimes, your doctor cannot tell which type of atrial flutter you have until measurements of the inside of your heart are made during an electrophysiology (EP) study. Many patients can be considered candidates for an ablation of atrial flutter during the first episode. It is important to talk to your doctor about the risks, benefits, and alternatives to considering ablation for atrial flutter. Of note, the ablation for typical atrial flutter is generally considered less risky than an ablation for atrial fibrillation. Moreover, atrial flutter can be cured, whereas atrial fibrillation is generally considered not curable, although ablation can significantly reduce the symptoms caused by atrial fibrillation. Appendix 3 helps explain the difference between atrial flutter and atrial fibrillation.

Common Clinical Scenario 4

A sixty-three-year-old man with a past medical history of obesity, hypertension, obstructive sleep apnea (untreated), and tobacco use was referred for evaluation of atrial fibrillation. The patient was doing well on metoprolol and flecainide. He reported one to two hours of mildly symptomatic atrial fibrillation that occurred every one to two weeks, mainly at bedtime. These symptoms did not disrupt his activities of daily living, and he was comfortable with his symptom burden. We talked about his level of symptoms from atrial fibrillation as well as noninvasive means by which we could further reduce his symptoms: treatment for obstructive sleep apnea, regular exercise, weight loss, tobacco cessation, and more aggressive blood pressure control. At the end of our visit, the patient decided to continue his current medical regimen and attempt the noninvasive measures described. Several months later, the patient appeared in my office with a cough severe enough that he could not complete full sentences. Since our last visit, he had been evaluated by another electrophysiologist who recommended an ablation for his atrial fibrillation. The patient underwent a cryoablation and suffered damage to his respiratory system from the procedure. The patient reported feeling worse than he did before the ablation, with no change in the frequency of atrial fibrillation. This is a powerful example of the importance of listening to the patient to assess severity of symptoms and counseling patients on the risks, benefits, and alternatives of procedures.

Summary. Atrial fibrillation is a very common arrhythmia encountered in cardiology and its prevalence is increasing as the population ages. We are still trying to understand the electrical causes of atrial fibrillation but it is clear that many patients with atrial fibrillation can have their symptoms reduced with both lifestyle interventions as well as medications and possible ablation. The most significant risk of atrial fibrillation is stroke, and the first step in treatment is deciding what type of anticoagulation is appropriate for your situation. Aspirin alone may be adequate, but you may require warfarin or one of the newer oral anticoagulants. You must realize that atrial fibrillation will not be completely treated (or understood) in a single visit. It is important to be an active participant in managing your atrial fibrillation with your care provider.

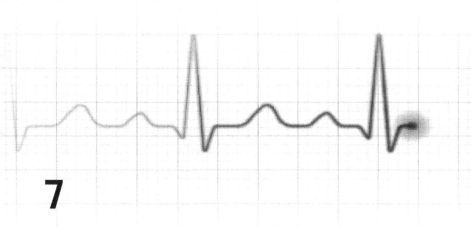

7

What Are the Common Ventricular (Bottom-Chamber) Tachycardias?

Premature ventricular contractions. Premature ventricular contractions (PVCs; also called ventricular premature contractions [VPCs] or ventricular premature depolarizations [VPD]) are extra signals from the bottom chambers (ventricles) that can trigger an extra heartbeat that interrupts the regular rhythm. As shown in figure 4A in chapter 2, PVCs may occur in over half of patients over sixty-five years of age. They are very common and generally harmless, although they may cause symptoms if they occur frequently. Studies have shown that when more than approximately 1 percent of heartbeats in a twenty-four-hour period are PVCs, a person's risk of death or heart failure increases; patients who have PVCs this frequently are often placed on medications called beta-blockers, such as atenolol, metoprolol, or carvedilol. Unless a patient develops heart failure from excessive numbers of PVCs (usually more than ten thousand in a twenty-four-hour period), the most appropriate treatment at this time is reassurance and possibly beta-blocker medications. In rare circumstances, an EP study may be recommended to ablate the PVC focus.

Ventricular tachycardia. Ventricular tachycardia (VT) is an arrhythmia that occurs when the bottom chambers of the heart (the ventricles) beat very rapidly. *Nonsustained* VT lasts for less than thirty seconds, and *sustained* VT lasts for more than thirty seconds. Most people who are diagnosed with VT have underlying heart disease that is usually due to coronary-artery disease. As discussed in chapter 2, it is important for patients to know their ejection fraction (EF). Asymptomatic nonsustained VT in patients with normal EFs (EF greater than 55–60 percent) generally does not portend higher death rates; these patients may not require any special treatment. Patients who have symptoms of VT (sustained or nonsustained) and patients with reduced EFs who have VT are usually prescribed beta-blockers; these types of patients may also have an EP study as part of their recommended treatment plan. Furthermore, calcium-channel blockers (diltiazem or verapamil) may be used in patients who cannot tolerate beta-blockers or in whom beta-blockers were ineffective. Figure 7D in chapter 5 shows an example of VT; note that at the end of the EKG, the VT stops, and the normal rhythm resumes. VT is differentiated from arrhythmias from the upper chambers (SVTs) by the wide QRS. Appendix 2 helps explain the mechanism of VT and how it differs from atrial tachycardia.

Common Clinical Scenario 5

A forty-seven-year-old female with no significant past medical history presented with palpitations from nonsustained ventricular tachycardia found on Holter monitoring. Echocardiogram, stress test (normal exercise capacity but possible perfusion defect on imaging), cardiac catheterization, and cardiac magnetic resonance imaging [MRI] revealed no significant structural heart disease. She opted for medical therapy with metoprolol and did well for over a year, with no recurrent symptoms. Ultimately, she presented with recurrent symptoms of palpitations and was found to have runs of ventricular tachycardia lasting ten to twenty seconds, and her ECG suggested right-ventricular outflow tract ventricular tachycardia (RVOT VT). She underwent an EP study and successful ablation for RVOT VT, with subsequent resolution of symptoms.

Non–coronary disease VT. Non–coronary disease VT occurs in less than 1 percent of patients. RVOT VT and left-ventricular outflow tract (LVOT) VT are types of ventricular tachycardias that occur in the pulmonary and aortic outflow tracts. The outflow tracts are the areas where blood flows out of the heart to the lungs (pulmonary outflow) or to the rest of the body (aortic outflow). Both RVOT and LVOT can be treated with medications but are often treated with EP studies and curative ablation. It is important to talk about these options with your care providers. Arrhythmogenic right- and left-ventricular dysplasia (AR/L/VD) VT are quite rare and can lead to sudden death. Patients with AR/L/VD are usually treated with both medications and defibrillators.

Common Clinical Scenario 6

A sixty-eight-year-old male with no significant past medical history reported that he was exercising on a treadmill and noticed that his heart rate continued to be elevated thirty minutes after stopping exercise. He presented to the emergency room and was found to be in sustained ventricular tachycardia that required cardioversion to return to his normal rhythm. Echocardiogram did not indicate any worrisome findings except mild right-ventricular wall motion abnormality, and cardiac catheterization did not reveal any obstructive coronary disease or heart failure. His signal-averaged electrocardiogram was mildly abnormal. He was placed on beta-blockers, and a wearable defibrillator was recommended to allow him to obtain a cardiac MRI (my hospital at the time did not have the ability to perform cardiac MRIs). The cardiac MRI confirmed a diagnosis of arrhythmogenic right-ventricular dysplasia (ARVD), and a defibrillator was successfully implanted. The patient was advised to no longer participate in vigorous exercise because this has been linked to progression of ARVD.

What are defibrillators? The easiest rule to remember is this: defibrillators are used to prevent the recurrence of a life-threatening ventricular arrhythmia (secondary prevention) or to avoid the initial occurrence of a life-threatening ventricular arrhythmia (primary prevention).

The decision to recommend a defibrillator requires an evaluation of the duration of the heart condition and whether or not the patient has been adequately treated for it; for example, has the patient been placed on the appropriate medications, and have coronary-artery blockages and other reversible causes of heart failure been addressed? Also, there are some diseases that may warrant defibrillator implantation even without the presence of heart failure (e.g., hypertrophic cardiomyopathy, long-QT syndrome, and arrhythmogenic right-ventricular dysplasia). Some patients may not be candidates for defibrillators because they cannot adequately follow up on device care or because their psychiatric conditions may be worsened by device implantations. Defibrillators are not appropriate for patients who have a life expectancy of less than one year. There is also a wearable, temporary defibrillator that is a temporary alternative to implantable defibrillators.

Not all occurrences of ventricular tachycardia are life threatening, and many do not require consideration of an implantable defibrillator. If you have been diagnosed with VT, it is important to discuss the type of VT and treatment options that may be available.

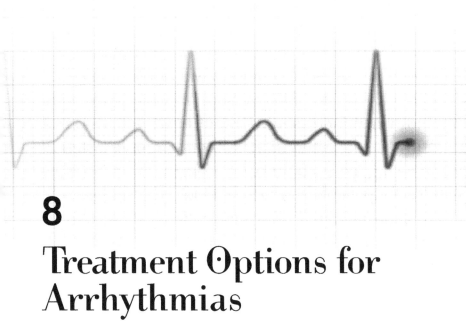

8
Treatment Options for Arrhythmias

Lifestyle. There are plenty of ways that patients can minimize the burden of arrhythmia without the use of procedures or medications. A *heart-healthy diet and lifestyle* is the first step toward reducing the risk of arrhythmia. Not only can a heart-healthy diet help with weight loss, but a proper diet can reduce the overall level of inflammation in your body, which can in turn decrease help decrease the risk of heart-rhythm abnormalities. *Regular exercise* (even walking) can help with weight loss as well as reduce the occurrence of heart-rhythm disorders. There is evidence that cardiovascular fitness can help reduce the occurrence of arrhythmia (including atrial fibrillation), although the mechanism and degree of this effect are unclear. Tobacco use (even smokeless as well as vaporized inhalants) can increase the inflammatory milieu in your body and hence increase the risk of heart-rhythm problems. *Tobacco cessation* is an important first step in reducing the occurrence of heart-rhythm problems. I had a patient who was scheduled to undergo an ablation for atrial fibrillation when he decided to quit smoking. He reduced his episodes of atrial fibrillation by over 80 percent, and we canceled his ablation because his symptoms had improved so much! Stress can be a powerful trigger for heart-rhythm problems, and *stress relief* can help reduce the occurrence of arrhythmias. Stress relief can take the form of exercise, relaxation methods like yoga, and even reading. Contrary to what many smokers think, tobacco cessation causes a reduction in stress! Some arrhythmias respond to *vagal maneuvers*. Vagal maneuvers are actions that stimulate the vagus nerve and slow the heart rate and include things like bearing down as if you were having a bowel movement, coughing vigorously, and placing your face in a bowl of ice water. These maneuvers cause your heart to slow conduction through the AV node and may terminate an arrhythmia. Vagal maneuvers are effective for some arrhythmias that use the heart's AV-node conduction system (see chapter 1, figure 2). However, these maneuvers don't always work and may not have any effect on certain types of arrhythmias; vagal maneuvers are generally ineffective for atrial fibrillation, atrial flutter, and ventricular arrhythmias. You should discuss vagal maneuvers with your doctor before attempting them at home.

Can exercise cause heart-rhythm problems? There is some evidence that extreme endurance training, such as for marathons, may increase the risk of atrial fibrillation; clearly, this does not apply to many patients. Generally, thirty to sixty minutes of vigorous exercise daily is adequate to reap the benefits of exercise. Another patient of mine had bouts of atrial fibrillation when training for triathlons; when he backed down to more reasonable levels of exercise, his burden of atrial fibrillation decreased tremendously (although not completely).

Medications. Each patient responds to each medication in a different manner. It is important to remember that not all patients have the same side effects to each medication. Any symptom that occurs after a new medication is started could be caused by that particular medicine. If you are concerned that a medication may be causing symptoms, please contact the prescribing provider. *If you develop a rash and/or difficulty breathing or swallowing after a new medicine is taken, stop the medicine immediately, and contact your doctor or call 911.*

Intravenous medications can be used emergently in an ambulance, in the emergency room, or in the hospital. Adenosine is a common intravenous medication that can be used to halt certain arrhythmias. It is a short-lasting medication that can cause a brief period of uncomfortable symptoms and may abruptly return the patient to a normal heart rhythm. Patients may also be given intravenous beta blockers or calcium channel blockers as well as a special medication called amiodarone.

Oral medications are commonly used to treat and prevent heart rhythm problems at home or while in the hospital. *Calcium-channel blockers* (CCBs), such as verapamil and diltiazem, can help slow the conduction of the native conduction system and reduce symptoms from arrhythmias. Common side effects of CCBs include fluid retention, constipation, and lowered blood pressure. *Beta-blockers,* such as atenolol, metoprolol, carvedilol, and propranolol, can also reduce the symptoms associated with heart rhythm abnormalities. Side effects of beta-blockers can include fatigue, slow heart rates, and upset stomach. Beta-blockers may not be appropriate for patients with severe lung disease. *Digoxin* has been around a long time and is sometimes used to treat arrhythmias. Side effects of digoxin may include nausea, dizziness, and vision changes. Patients with kidney disease should be cautious using digoxin.

Not every patient responds to these medications the same way, and each patient may have different side effects from a given medication. If you are having possible side effects from a medication, talk to your doctor immediately.

The Vaughan-Williams Classification (Classes 1, 2, 3, and 4) is a system used to classify *antiarrhythmics* based on their mechanism of action. Table 5 describes the different classes of antiarrhythmics and how they are used, as well as side effects. I will briefly cover some of the more common agents I use in my practice.

Table 5. The Vaughan-Williams Classification (Classes 1, 2, 3, and 4)

Vaughan-Williams Class	Medications	How It Is Used	Side Effects
1 (Sodium-Channel Blockers)	Flecainide, procainamide, disopyramide, quinidine	Atrial fibrillation, accessory pathways, ventricular arrhythmias	Can cause arrhythmias, dry mouth, decreased heart contractility, and ECG abnormalities
2 (Beta Blockers)	Metoprolol, carvedilol, propranolol, atenolol, bisoprolol	Heart attacks, coronary-artery blockages, heart failure	Can make you feel lethargic or dizzy; may lower blood pressure and heart rate; should not be stopped abruptly
3 (Potassium-Channel Blockers)	Amiodarone, sotalol, ibutilide, dofetilide, dronedarone	Atrial and ventricular arrhythmias	Can cause arrhythmias, fatigue, and ECG abnormalities
4 (Calcium-Channel Blockers)	Verapamil, diltiazem	Atrial arrhythmias	Can cause constipation and lower extremity swelling

ECG=electrocardiogram.

Flecainide and propafenone are Class 1C medications in the Vaughan-Williams system and are generally my first-line antiarrhythmics in patients who don't have structural heart disease; they are especially useful for atrial fibrillation. Class 1C categorizes antiarrhythmics based on their ion-channel mechanism of action; detailed discussion of this system is beyond the scope of this book. Patients without structural heart disease include younger patients who don't have heart disease caused by high blood pressure (which results in significant left-ventricular hypertrophy), heart failure (with reduced ejection fraction), or prior heart attack. These medications are usually used with calcium-channel blockers and beta-blockers to prevent potentially dangerous fast heart rates.

Amiodarone (Class 3) is the most effective medication for atrial fibrillation and ventricular arrhythmias. It also has the most side effects of all antiarrhythmics; 60 percent of patients have amiodarone discontinued within two years because of adverse side effects. These side effects include sun sensitivity, nausea, tremors, and thyroid and pulmonary problems. Amiodarone can be safely started on an outpatient basis and does not require hospitalization. This medicine is stored in fat cells and can take several weeks to wear off once a patient stops taking it.

Dronedarone (Class 3) is a close relative of amiodarone but does not include iodine as part of its chemical makeup. Theoretically, this lack of iodine causes less side effects, but this medicine can cause side effects similar to those of amiodarone. It can be safely started as an outpatient but should not be used in patients with permanent atrial fibrillation or recent episodes of heart failure.

Sotalol (Class 3) can be a very effective medicine against atrial fibrillation and, less commonly, ventricular arrhythmias. It generally requires several days of hospitalization when it is started to make sure the medication does not trigger a dangerous (and thankfully very rare) arrhythmia. This medicine is taken twice daily, and once five doses have been safely administered in the hospital setting, the patient can then continue taking this medicine at home. Changes in kidney function can result in changes in the medicine dose or require discontinuation. Similar to beta-blockers, sotalol can cause malaise, fatigue, abnormally slow heart rates (bradycardia), and shortness of breath.

Dofetilide (Class 3) can also be a very effective medicine against atrial fibrillation and ventricular arrhythmias. Like sotalol, it requires several days of hospitalization when it is started to make sure the medication does not trigger a dangerous (and thankfully very rare) arrhythmia. This medicine is taken twice daily, and once five doses haven been safely administered in the hospital setting, the patient can then continue taking this medicine at home. Changes in kidney function can result in changes in medicine dose or require discontinuation. Medicines such as cimetidine, hydrochlorothiazide, triamterene, antifungals, trimethoprim/sulfamethoxazole, or verapamil cannot be taken with this medicine. Dofetilide is generally well tolerated, but patients could experience dizziness, stomach issues, or slow heart rates.

Anticoagulation. Anticoagulation may be an important element of arrhythmia treatment, especially with atrial fibrillation and atrial flutter. You should discuss your risk of stroke and anticoagulation options with your care provider.

Ablation. Ablation is a means to treat arrhythmias by delivering very precise burns to the inside of your heart. Small catheters are placed in the femoral veins of your legs (where the inguinal crease is located) and advanced into your heart. These catheters are then used to diagnose the abnormality and, if possible, deliver electrical energy to burn the inside of your heart to eradicate the abnormal areas that are responsible for the abnormal heart rhythms. See chapters 9 and 10 for more information about ablation.

Cardioversion. Cardioversion is a way to return your heart rhythm to its normal (sinus) rhythm. Chemical cardioversion uses medicine to terminate an abnormal heart rhythm. Chemical cardioversion can be performed with ibutilide, amiodarone, flecainide, propafenone, or procainamide. Electrical cardioversion uses an electrical shock (delivered with paddles or, more commonly, adhesive patches placed on the chest over the heart) to terminate an abnormal heart rhythm. Both chemical and electrical cardioversions are performed in a hospital setting, and the patient is gently sedated to prevent discomfort. There are special situations where a patient can take a dose of flecainide or propafenone while not in the hospital (called the *pill-in-pocket* regimen) to terminate atrial fibrillation; this pill-in-pocket method is usually performed under the direction of cardiologists or electrophysiologists and is usually first performed in a hospital setting.

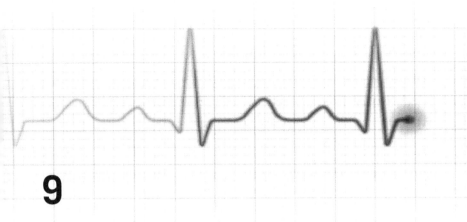

9

The Electrophysiology Study and Ablation Procedure

If medicines and lifestyle modifications are ineffective at relieving abnormal heart rhythms, your doctor may recommend an electrophysiology (EP) study and possible ablation. An EP study is a test of the electrical systems of your heart. It is usually done because you have had symptoms that indicate that your heart may occasionally be beating too fast.

You will need to come to an EP laboratory (which is very similar to the special laboratory where heart catheterizations are performed to look for blockages in coronary arteries) to have this procedure done. The doctor will insert large intravenous sheaths (hollow tubes) into one or more of your big veins, usually in the groin but possibly at other sites. The sheaths will be used by the doctor to thread special catheters into specific areas inside your heart. With these catheters, the doctor will evaluate the electrical system of your heart. The doctor may also try to cause your particular type of abnormal heartbeat so that he or she can see where it comes from and what makes it happen. If the doctor is successful in causing the abnormal heartbeat to occur, he or she may be able to demonstrate the same arrhythmia that was recorded in the outpatient setting. If the doctor is able to find a specific source for your abnormal heartbeat, he or she will steer a catheter to the spot in your heart that is triggering the arrhythmia. The doctor will advance the catheter to the identified spot and put a tiny burn (called *ablation*) on it with a special type of energy called *radiofrequency* (high-energy sound waves) or *cryoablation* (using supercool temperatures to freeze the areas). More than one application of energy is often needed. To get the catheter to the spot causing the abnormal rhythm, the doctor may need to put a tiny hole in the membrane that divides the two upper chambers of the heart to reach the left side of the heart (called a *transseptal puncture*).

Questions to Ask Your Doctor before an EP Study or Ablation

1. What is your training background?

There is evidence that physician training (specifically, board certification or board eligibility in clinical cardiac electrophysiology) may result in lower rates of complications (Cheng et al. 2010; Curtis et al. 2009).

2. How many EP studies/ablations have you done?

Doctors who have performed more ablations seem to have fewer complications than doctors with less experience.

3. What complications have you seen?

This question can be especially enlightening because it will give you an idea of whether the doctor has looked at his or her outcomes. A doctor who tells you that he or she has had no complications is misinformed or has not done enough procedures. Any doctor who performs procedures has complications, and a doctor who cares about patient outcomes will have

> *done due diligence to minimize complications from happening again. That being said, there is generally no way to have no complications, but it is important to choose a doctor who has in-depth knowledge of possible complications.*

Preoperative risk assessment. As with all surgical procedures, recognizing and managing existing medical problems (aka comorbid conditions) preoperatively helps to mitigate the risks during and immediately after EP studies. Many patients undergoing EP studies have heart failure, structural heart disease, and/or disease of the cardiac conduction system, which means that there is an inherently high-risk population of patients frequently served in the EP lab. Indeed, congestive heart failure (CHF) increases the risk of all surgery. A decreased ejection fraction has been found to be a predictor of perioperative complications, with the highest-risk group being those with an EF less than 35 percent. Preprocedural management of CHF is integral to the safety of the procedure. Patients certainly should not be in a state of decompensated heart failure.

Use of contrast agents during EP studies or ablations (Williams and Stevenson 2012). Bones show up very well on x-rays; however, soft structures such as blood vessels and the heart do not. Therefore, blood vessels and heart structure are highlighted by *contrast,* a clear liquid designed for use during EP studies or ablations. The doctor may use fluoroscopy to guide the procedure. Fluoroscopy is a special type of imaging that allows the doctor to perform x-rays while the patient or the heart is moving. Fluoroscopy allows doctors to watch catheters and leads moving in the blood vessels and the heart so that we can place them in the correct location. A typical use of contrast for an EP study is during an ablation that is close to one of the coronary arteries (this is not very common). Coronary arteriography is done to ensure that a patient's coronary artery is not near where we plan to perform an ablation; delivering ablative energy near a coronary artery can lead to a blockage. If we feel we are too close to a coronary artery, we can change the location of the catheter, or we may opt to stop the procedure.

Contrast-induced nephropathy (CIN). Contrast-induced nephropathy (kidney failure) is a surprisingly common complication if radiocontrast is given during a procedure; CIN can occur in 15 percent of cases. It is a decline in kidney function (assessed by checking the blood level of creatinine) that typically peaks at forty-eight to seventy-two hours after exposure. Creatinine may remain above baseline for seven to fourteen days. Naturally, the best way to avoid this complication is to abstain from the use of contrast.

Thankfully, we generally do not require much (if any) contrast during most EP studies and ablations. However, many patients undergoing EP studies are patients with heart failure and its associated comorbidities—which frequently include diabetes and chronic kidney disease. Therefore, a working knowledge of and respect for these agents is a necessity. There are several things I may do to limit the danger of kidney damage; they include (1) using a very weak, diluted contrast agent; (2) aggressively hydrating the patient (especially one with kidney disease at baseline; hydration can usually be achieved with four to six glasses of water the evening before the procedure); and (3) holding medications that can worsen kidney damage during the procedure (e.g., angiotensin-converting enzyme [ACE] inhibitors, angiotensin-receptor blockers, and nonsteroidal anti-inflammatory drugs [NSAIDS] can be held the day prior and day of exposure and be resumed twenty-four hours after exposure, and medications such as sodium bicarbonate and N-acetylcysteine [Mucomyst] can be given prior to the procedure). Treatment of CIN is largely supportive (generally resolves on its own) and infrequently requires short-term dialysis.

Contrast allergies. Immediate life-threatening allergic (anaphylactic) reactions—including angioedema (face and throat swelling), bronchospasm (lung spasm), arterial hypotension (low blood pressure), and shock—can occur within minutes of and up to sixty minutes after injection of intravenous (IV) contrast (Marcos and Thomsen 2001). The reported incidence of severe immediate reactions to ionic contrast material is 0.1 to 0.4 percent, and with the newer, nonionic, and low-osmolar or iso-osmolar contrast, it is 0.02 to 0.04 percent. But death rates from the two materials do not differ (Brockow et al. 2005). Patients with even mild anaphylactoid (immediate) reactions should be considered high-risk patients in future procedures involving contrast administration.

It is common practice to premedicate with corticosteroids with or without histamine (H1) blockers (e.g., Pepcid) in patients with histories of moderate or severe immediate reactions, despite the fact that randomized trials comparing pretreatment strategies are severely lacking. Prior to any procedure that may involve contrast administration, *it is essential that you inform your doctor about any history of previous contrast reaction, asthma, renal insufficiency, diabetes, and metformin therapy* (Royal College of Radiologists 2010). Routine premedication of all patients who receive contrast is probably not warranted given the overall low incidence of a reaction; in fact, some have advocated abandoning this procedure (Tramer et al. 2006). Patients with a history of severe contrast allergy who will likely need IV contrast during a procedure should probably receive preexposure treatment with corticosteroids (such as prednisone or hydrocortisone) as well as H1 blockers, although strong evidence of benefit is lacking (Trcka et al. 2008). If contrast administration cannot be delayed for four to six hours after steroids, some doctors will omit steroid use and administer only H1 blockers (Royal College of Radiologists 2010). Weaker agents—such as low-osmolar or iso-osmolar contrast such as ioxaglate, iohexol, or ioversol—should be used due to the lower overall incidence of reactions in patients with a history of asthma or a contrast allergy. The specific contrast agent causing the prior reaction should be sought and avoided if possible, although this information is often difficult for your doctor to obtain. Despite pretreatment with steroids and H1 blockers, reactions are still possible in those with prior reactions.

Thyroid issues (Williams and Stevenson 2012). Hypothyroidism (low thyroid function) has been found in 0.5 to 0.8 percent of the population; it is demonstrated by elevated serum levels of thyroid-stimulating hormone (TSH) or decreased serum thyroxine levels (Murkin 1982). Undiagnosed (hence, untreated) hypothyroidism can lead to major perioperative complications, including severe hypotension (low blood pressure) or cardiac arrest following induction of anesthesia; extreme sensitivity to narcotics and anesthetics, with prolonged unconsciousness; and hypothyroid coma following anesthesia and surgery (Murkin 1982). Ideally, hypothyroidism is caught early in the preoperative evaluation, and a thyroid supplement (thyroxine) may be administered until the patient's thyroid function has normalized—generally in four to six weeks.

Hyperthyroidism (high thyroid function) affects approximately 0.2 percent of men and 2 percent of women and may cause atrial fibrillation, congestive heart failure, and a reduction in the number of blood cells (called thrombocytopenia) (Farling 2000). In addition, anesthetic drugs may be affected by the hypermetabolic state of hyperthyroidism. When total IV anesthesia is used, an increased dose of sedatives may be needed because these agents are processed more quickly with a hyperactive thyroid (Farling 2000; Williams et al. 2011). In my practice at the Heart Rhythm Center, this may occur when high-frequency ventilation is used to minimize respiratory motion during heart procedures.

Generally, more thyroid-related perioperative complications stem from hypothyroidism as opposed to hyperthyroidism; however, recognition of either condition prior to implantation is important. At the Heart Rhythm Center, we usually obtain TSH prior to EP studies, and we often allow four to six weeks for the patient's thyroid function to normalize prior to proceeding with surgery. Emergent cases with thyroid abnormalities require close coordination with anesthesiology and will generally be undertaken with general anesthesia.

Allergies. Obviously, your doctors should be aware of any drug allergy or prior concerning reaction to any medication. The first exposure to a medication often causes a minor reaction, but the second exposure can lead to a fatal allergic reaction called *anaphylaxis*. It is also important to let your doctor know if you have had any reactions to other substances. Knowledge of a prior reaction to IV contrast agents (such as during a computed tomography [CT] scan or cardiac catheterization) or latex gloves can enable your doctors to avoid using these agents or give preventive medications (called *prophylaxis*) so that an adverse reaction is minimized. Prophylaxis may include the use of steroids and antihistamines. Steroids such as prednisone and hydrocortisone are often used preoperatively. In addition, antihistamines such as diphenhydramine (Benadryl) and famotidine (Pepcid) are given to reduce the severity of a possible allergic reaction.

Registration and check-in. Patients generally undergo EP studies at the hospital and require an overnight stay. Rarely do patients go home the same day as an EP study that includes an ablation, although this can happen. Some doctors operate at multiple hospitals, so it is important to verify the hospital at which the procedure is to be done. The patient will generally check in with registration and then go to the appropriate *holding area* (preoperative or "preop" unit). This is a staging area where the patient changes into a gown, an IV is started, and hospital documentation is performed. Prior to the procedure, the patient is asked multiple times to state his or her name and the type of procedure that is to be performed. Questions often seem redundant (e.g., Do you have any allergies? What surgery are you here for?) but this fact-checking process is an attempt to minimize any chance of medical error. Many doctors will meet their patients in the holding area to answer any last-minute questions and confirm that all preoperative tests are complete and the surgery can proceed.

Informed-consent process. The informed-consent process is one of the most important aspects of any medical procedure. It is more than just getting a patient to sign the consent form. This is the process by which a patient is informed of the diagnosis and the nature and purpose of the proposed treatment or procedure. The patient should understand the risks and benefits of the proposed EP study as well as the risks and benefits of any alternative treatments, such as medications or watchful waiting. This book can be part of the informed-consent process because it covers all aspects of arrhythmia evaluation in a more thorough manner than can be presented in even multiple office visits. It is during this process that patients can make sure they fully understand the rationales for their EP studies and can ask any questions they might have for the physician. Some physicians go over these risks, benefits, and alternatives in the office and have their patients more thoroughly review and read the consent form at home prior to surgery. Once the patient has completed the required elements in the holding area and the informed-consent process is completed, he or she is brought into the *procedure room.*

The procedure room. The procedure room may be a standard operating room or may be a specialized cardiac-catheterization laboratory (where heart catheterizations are usually performed) that has been altered to perform EP studies. A *time-out* (once the patient is in the procedure room) occurs when the doctors, nurses, technologists, and all other personnel who are participating in the surgery stop what they are doing (before the patient is sedated) and identify the patient, the procedure being performed (including site of implant), the technique to be used, and any other important patient information (such as drug allergies). The time-out is usually performed to minimize the occurrence of any medical errors—such as performing an EP study in the wrong patient!

At this point, the procedure can be started. Most patients are sedated for the EP study. Conscious sedation involves giving medications that relax the patient and relieve pain but allow the patient to breathe on his or her own. Conscious sedation can be administered by nurses in the room or by anesthesiologists. General anesthesia involves deep sedation, and it often requires a temporary breathing tube and a connection to an artificial ventilator. General anesthesia is administered by anesthesiologists or specially trained nurses called *certified registered nurse anesthetists* (CRNAs). The higher the risk of the surgery, the more often general anesthesia is used. General anesthesia may permit tighter control of patient heart rate and blood pressure and allow the patient to remain absolutely still during the procedure. These elements may permit a safer procedure as well as a more pleasant experience for the patient.

The EP study. The EP study is performed in an operating room or cardiac procedure room that includes sterile supplies, an adjustable patient table, and an x-ray system called fluoroscopy. Figure 8 shows a typical EP procedure room. The C-arm holds the x-ray equipment that the physician uses to guide the catheters into their correct positions; this technique of using x-rays to guide catheter placement is called fluoroscopy. The screens display patient information—such as EKG and blood pressure—and show the x-ray images. The anesthesia equipment and anesthesiologist are at the head of the bed. A special sterile table holds all the instruments and equipment that will be used during the EP study.

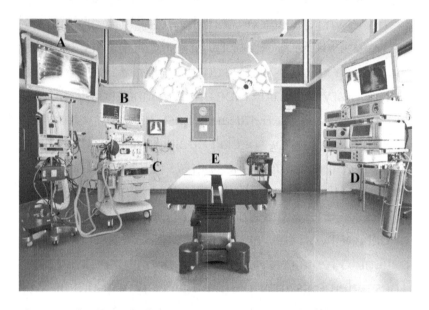

Figure 8. The EP Procedure Room. This is a dedicated EP procedure room that includes (A) x-ray equipment to guide catheter placement, (B) screens displaying patient information, (C) anesthesia equipment, (D) testing equipment, and (E) the patient table.

The EP study usually involves placing multiple catheters in the femoral veins. These are the large veins found in the groin creases. Your doctor may also place a catheter in a femoral artery to monitor blood pressure and, rarely, place a catheter in the artery to access certain parts of your heart not easily reached via the veins. Catheters are sometimes placed in the large veins of your neck (internal jugular). These veins lead to your heart.

Operative Steps of EP Studies

1. Sterile preparation and draping of the patient occur on the operating table.

2. The patient is sedated.

3. Specialized personnel prepare the right or left groin and cover the rest of the patient with sterile gowns.

4. The EP physician washes his or her hands and then puts on a sterile gown and gloves.

5. Lidocaine is used to numb the skin where vascular access will be placed. These sites are usually in the femoral veins located in the creases of your groin.

6. The femoral vein (and sometimes artery) is punctured with a needle, and a wire is placed through this needle. The needle is withdrawn — leaving the wire in the blood vessel. Over this wire, a hollow tube (called a sheath) is placed, and a catheter that can measure electrical activity is placed through this sheath. This is repeated for each catheter the doctor needs to place into your heart.

7. Once the doctor places all the necessary sheaths and catheters into your heart, the doctor begins to make baseline electrical measurements of your heart's conduction system.

8. After the baseline measurements are obtained, the doctor will then use special pacing maneuvers in an attempt to cause an arrhythmia. Hopefully, the induced arrhythmia is the same one you experienced at home.

9. The vascular access, baseline measurements, and arrhythmia induction may take several hours. Ultimately, an ablation may be performed. The entire EP study and ablation may take as long as four to six hours.

10. The catheters are then withdrawn from your heart, the sheaths are removed, manual pressure is applied to stop bleeding, and the patient is awakened from sedation and returned to the recovery area.

How does the doctor place catheters inside the heart? The doctor uses a special real-time x-ray system (called fluoroscopy) to position the EP catheters inside your heart via your veins. Figure 9 shows a fluoroscopic view of the heart during an EP study. Electrophysiologists complete many years of training to learn how to carefully place these catheters.

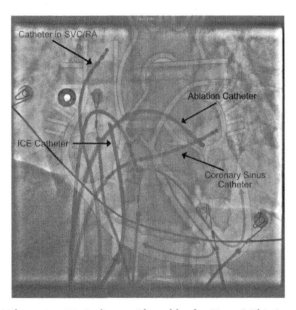

Figure 9. Where Are EP Catheters Placed in the Heart? This is a typical fluoroscopic image (a special type of chest x-ray)—with a superimposed cartoon of the heart to show the *approximate* location of the cardiac chambers—used to verify catheter placement. Your cardiologist uses this imaging to make sure that the catheters are in the correct chamber of the heart. The intracardiac echocardiographic (ICE) catheter is used to visualize the inside of your heart and guide the placement of the other EP catheters.

What happens if my doctor cannot successfully find an arrhythmia? This sometimes happens, although it is disappointing for both you and your doctor. On the one hand, if we couldn't find the arrhythmia, it is usually reassuring that we are not dealing with a particularly dangerous arrhythmia. On the other hand, the patient may still experience symptoms once he or she is back at home. I usually try to "demonstrate" the arrhythmia before subjecting a patient to an EP study; that is, we try various types of home monitoring to record an arrhythmia that is causing the symptoms. If we are unable to capture an arrhythmia on some type of home monitoring, it is more likely that we won't be able to cause (or *induce*) an arrhythmia during an EP study.

What happens if my doctor cannot successfully ablate the arrhythmia? Unsuccessful ablation attempts can also be disappointing. Some arrhythmias can be caused in the EP lab, but despite multiple attempts, they cannot be successfully pinpointed and ablated. This could be due to several factors: patient movement, an arrhythmia focus on the outside wall of the heart, or an arrhythmia focus deep in the heart muscle. Sometimes, patients with AV-node reentrant tachycardia have an arrhythmia focus that is very close to the conduction system; placing burns too close to the native conduction system could cause complete heart block and necessitate pacemaker implantation. Figure 10 gives estimates on the success rates of ablations for some of the more common arrhythmias. Atrioventricular nodal reentrant tachycardia (AVNRT), atrioventricular reentrant tachycardia (AVRT), and typical atrial flutter tend to have high success rates (~95 percent single-procedure success rates). Success rates for ablation need to be balanced with the risks of complication for each type of ablation. Indeed, as discussed previously, ablations for atrial fibrillation and ventricular tachycardia (in patients with advanced coronary-artery disease) tend to have higher rates of complications and lower rates of successful ablations (~60–70 percent single-procedure success rates). Of patients undergoing an ablation for atrial fibrillation, approximately 15 percent of patients may require a repeat ablation within one year of the initial procedure, and approximately 30 percent of these patients will require a repeat ablation within three years of the initial procedure. Of patients undergoing an ablation for ventricular tachycardia, 60 percent will have recurrent ventricular tachycardia (VT) within six months of the initial procedure.

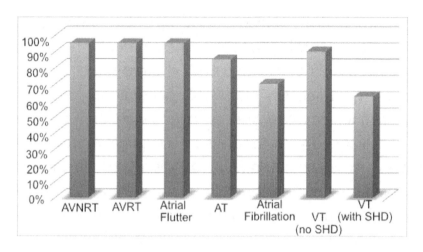

Figure 10. Estimated Single-Procedure Success Rates of Ablations for Various Arrhythmias. AVNRT=atrioventricular nodal reentrant tachycardia, AVRT=atrioventricular reentrant tachycardia, AT=atrial tachycardia, VT=ventricular tachycardia, SHD=structural heart disease (e.g., coronary-artery disease). (Adapted from Williams et al. 2010 and Tung, Boyle, and Shivkumar 2010.)

Immediately after the EP study. Once the patient is awake, with no obvious complications, he or she is generally observed in the hospital overnight, although some centers may offer to send patients home the same day. The doctor will usually talk to the patient and his or her family about the procedure. The discussion with family or friends is important; the patient may not remember events in the immediate postoperative period because of the sedatives given during the procedure. At the Heart Rhythm Center, our patients are generally kept lying in bed for four to six hours after the EP study. They can eat once they are awake and alert after the procedure. We keep a sterile dressing on the vascular access sites until the next morning when we examine the area.

Day after the EP study. The morning after the EP study, the vascular access sites are inspected by the doctor, a nurse, or an assistant. Generally, the incision can be left without a gauze dressing—as long as the incision-care instructions in next section are followed. If there is any oozing, clean, dry gauze can be placed over the incision to protect clothing from blood staining. Once the vascular access sites are found to be healthy, the patient is ready to go home. The electrophysiologist may not see the patient the day after the EP study, but the physician's team will be very familiar with care following an EP study and the process of arranging discharge from the hospital. Please note that some EP studies and ablations (such as those for atrial fibrillation or ventricular tachycardia) may require a patient to stay in the hospital for more than one night.

Advanced treatment options for atrial fibrillation. Sometimes medications may not be enough to control symptoms from atrial fibrillation. If catheter ablation of atrial fibrillation is not sufficient to reduce symptoms, there are open heart surgery options (for example, a Maze procedure) that may be appropriate for some patients. If a patient is not considered a candidate for atrial fibrillation ablation, one of these surgical options and all else fails, an AV node ablation can be considered. This procedure prevents the atria from sending rapid electrical signals to the ventricles but atrial fibrillation continues. A pacemaker is then implanted so the ventricles continue to beat properly. After the AV node ablation and pacemaker implantation, your atria continue to fibrillate and anticoagulation to reduce the risk of stroke is still necessary. AV node ablation and pacemaker implantation can be a great option in elderly patients that have difficulty tolerating the medications (such as beta blockers and calcium channel blockers) used to control atrial fibrillation and slow the heart rates.

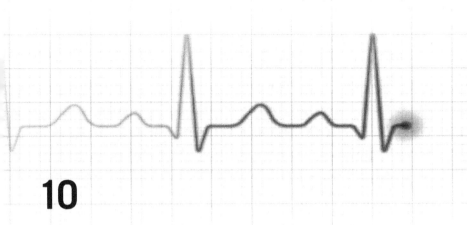

10

Possible Complications of Electrophysiology Studies and Ablations

Introduction. This section is written for both patients and primary-care doctors and is a bit more complex than the rest of the book. In most cases, I have attempted to boil the complication rates down to simple percentages. This section will familiarize patients with the names of common complications and how we detect and treat them.

Major and minor complications have been defined based on prior reports of complications related to anesthesia and electrophysiology (EP) procedures

(Hautmann et al. 2000; Hemmes et al. 2011; Jaquet et al. 2006; Williams et al. 2010). Major complications include death, cardiac arrest, AV block requiring a pacemaker, cardiac perforation, cardiac valve injury, coronary venous dissection, hemothorax, pneumothorax, transient ischemic attack, stroke, myocardial infarction, pericardial tamponade, severe respiratory failure, and acute respiratory distress syndrome. Minor complications include intraprocedural drug reaction, peripheral embolus, phlebitis, peripheral nerve injury, atelectasis, pulmonary edema, fever, and pleural effusion.

Prior reports indicate a *2 to 7 percent rate of major and minor complications during EP studies with ablation* using traditional sedation/ventilation methods (Chen et al. 1996; O'Hara et al. 2007; Williams et al. 2011; Zado et al. 2000). Many of these complications are minor (e.g., atelectasis, fever, vascular congestion, pericarditis) and generally do not prolong hospitalization. Closer examination of the results in my experience reveals that minor complications (e.g., atelectasis, fever, vascular congestion) may simply be reflective of common pulmonary complications seen after general anesthesia. Atelectasis can be seen on computed tomography

(CT) scan in up to 90 percent of patients who are anesthetized (Magnusson and Spahn 2003), and postoperative pulmonary complications have been found to occur in 9.6 percent of patients (Lawrence et al. 1995). Furthermore, 40 percent of the minor complications in a prior study of mine were related to atelectasis. *Atelectasis* is a minor collapse of the small airways in the lungs that is treated by deep breathing (called *incentive spirometry*). It is also important to note that no patient experienced procedural awareness during the procedure. Awareness with recall after surgery in the United States is infrequent (0.13–1.0 percent incidence) but may be associated with posttraumatic stress disorder in nearly 50 percent of patients who experience procedural awareness (Avidan et al. 2011; Sebel et al. 2004).

Finally, ablations for atrial fibrillation are considered higher risk than those for most other arrhythmias (excluding ventricular tachycardia). I estimate a *3 to 5 percent rate of major complications for patients undergoing atrial fibrillation ablations.* This is based on the overall, worldwide rate of complications for thousands of patients who underwent ablations for atrial fibrillation at centers around the world (Cappato et al. 2009). It must be noted that the major complication rates of atrial fibrillation (and ventricular tachycardia) ablation could be as high as 10 percent. Studies have found that clinicians often underestimate the rate of complications and overestimate the success rates of most medical interventions. It is important to talk to your care providers about the risks and benefits of any procedure that is being considered.

There is obviously a difference in complication rates based on the operating physician and the hospital in which the physician practices. I examined the complication rates of the first consecutive seventy-two EP studies with ablations performed when starting a new EP program at a community hospital (Williams et al. 2011). I did not have any major complications in this series of patients; however, I have had major complications in EP studies and ablations. It is important to note that past success rates do not guarantee future performance. All procedures have a risk of complications! See chapter 5 for the questions to ask your doctor before having surgery.

Complications that can occur during or after EP studies. The following sections describe the most common complications that can occur during or after EP studies.

Sedation/airway. Less than 20 percent of EP programs in the United States exclusively use anesthesia professionals for procedural sedation (Gaitan et al. 2011). Minor complications (e.g., atelectasis or minor lung compression, fever, or vascular congestion) may simply be reflective of the common postoperative pulmonary complications (PPCs) seen after general anesthesia. Atelectasis can be seen on CT scan in up to 90 percent of patients who are anesthetized (Magnusson and Spahn 2003), and PPCs have been found to occur in 9.6 percent of patients (Lawrence et al. 1995). There are data to suggest that patients undergoing invasive EP procedures may require deep conscious sedation that often is converted to general anesthesia (Trentman et al. 2009); thus, the use of general anesthesia (including high-frequency ventilation to minimize patient movement) during EP procedures may enhance patient safety (DiBiase et al. 2011; Williams et al. 2011).

Electrical heart block. Heart block may be caused when ablation is performed near the AV node in a patient during the EP study. This has been found to occur in as many as five out of every one hundred patients (Hindricks 1993); however, my experience has been that fewer than one in one hundred patients will experience permanent heart block requiring pacemaker implantation.

Vascular access and bleeding. Vascular access can be a significant cause of peri-procedural complications and may occur in up to 1 to 2 percent of patients after EP studies. A hematoma is a collection of blood outside the blood vessel but underneath the skin. The development of postoperative hematoma places the patient at elevated risk of infection (Sohail et al. 2011), especially if a device is implanted at the site. Most hematomas resolve with watchful waiting and do not require a surgical repair. They resolve over four to six weeks and can often have significant associated bruising, which also resolves over that time period. Worrisome signs include continued swelling, redness, warmth, bleeding, oozing, or changes in the incision. It is important to call your physician with any worries about incision or pocket healing.

Another type of vascular complications is a *pseudoaneurysm*; this forms as a result of a leaking hole in a blood vessel that allows blood to accumulate in surrounding tissue. Persistent communication between the blood vessel and the resultant cavity in the surrounding tissue can cause swelling and pain. This can often be treated by a radiologist placing pressure on the region using ultrasound guidance or injecting a medication called thrombin into the site to stop the bleeding, although surgery may be required in some circumstances. Finally, an *arteriovenous fistula* is a vascular complication in which an artery and vein develop an abnormal connection. Arteriovenous fistulas can be treated with ultrasound-guided compression but may require surgical repair. Either of these complications can cause swelling and pain at the site, and both are usually diagnosed by using ultrasound to look for abnormal blood collections or flow.

There are data to suggest that temporarily interrupting anticoagulation (e.g., stopping Coumadin) is associated with increased thromboembolic events (e.g., strokes or transient ischemic attacks), whereas cessation of warfarin with bridging anticoagulation with heparin products is associated with a higher rate of hematomas and a longer hospital stay (Ahmed et al. 2010). The issue of perioperative anticoagulation is very important to discuss with the doctor who will be performing your EP study. I routinely perform

EP studies while continuing warfarin uninterrupted. Patients who take target specific oral anticoagulants such as Xarelto, Eliquis, or Pradaxa need to talk with their doctor about whether or not these agents should be taken prior to the procedure. I generally have patients hold these medications for one to two days prior to the procedure and restart them one to three days after the procedure. No matter which vascular-access technique used, generally, the more experience a doctor has, the lower the complication rate.

Perforation/tamponade. Perforation occurs when trauma causes an unintended hole in a blood vessel or the walls of the heart; it can be a life-threatening situation. Perforation (both acute and subacute) has been reported to occur in up to 1 percent of EP studies and ablations (Zado et al. 2000). Symptoms of perforation include pleuritic chest pain from pericarditis and, in the presence of pericardial effusion (blood collecting around the outside of the heart), the possible development of shortness of breath and hypotension as tamponade develops (Wang et al. 2009). Tamponade occurs when enough blood collects on the outside of the heart that it can compress the heart and render it unable to pump blood effectively. Other signs/symptoms of perforation include electrocardiogram (EKG) abnormalities and friction rub (which sounds like rubbing sandpaper heard on stethoscope) after a procedure. If perforation is suspected, urgent evaluation of the patient is warranted; often, the first step is to check an echocardiogram of the heart to see if there is any blood collecting around the outside of the heart (called a pericardial effusion).

Cardiac surgery is typically not required for the majority of patients diagnosed with cardiac perforation caused during an EP study and ablation. Rather, most cases can be managed with pericardiocentesis (drainage of blood with a small catheter) performed by an interventional cardiologist for symptomatic effusions in the EP laboratory with close cardiothoracic surgical collaboration (Geyfman et al. 2007; Mahapatra 2005; Wang et al. 2009). Figure 11 shows a large cardiac silhouette—developing after pacemaker implantation—that was due to a large pericardial effusion. The effusion was treated with pericardiocentesis (with no evidence of blood reaccumulation). Although perforation and subsequent tamponade are infrequent complications of EP studies, they can be responsible for significant patient morbidity (any untoward side effect from a procedure) and mortality (death). The risks of perforation cannot be underestimated; death from tamponade with subsequent cardiac arrest was responsible for 21.8 percent of the deaths in a worldwide study of perforation after ablation for atrial fibrillation (Cappato et al. 2009).

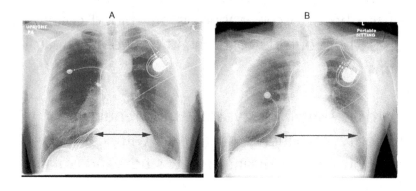

Figure 11. Chest Radiograph Appearance of Large Pericardial Effusion after Cardiac Perforation. (A) Immediately following the implantation of a pacemaker, the chest x-ray (CXR) shows a normal appearance of the cardiac silhouette. (B) At two weeks postoperative, the CXR (performed because the patient reported symptoms of chest pressure) shows an enlarged cardiac silhouette. The patient responded to pericardiocentesis with no lead repositioning. (Figure originally published by Williams and Stevenson 2012.)

Heart attacks. Heart attacks are also called *myocardial infarctions* (MIs) and are the most common cause of death after any surgery. They generally occur in less than 1 percent of EP studies. Again, the physician performing the EP study generally assesses the risk of surgery prior to the procedure, and patients at high risk of heart attacks may need additional heart care prior to proceeding with the EP study. *Keep in mind that those patients who have advanced coronary-artery disease causing heart failure with arrhythmias can be at the highest risk for perioperative heart attacks.*

Death. In-hospital death is very rare in patients undergoing EP studies and ablations except in the case of atrial fibrillation and ventricular tachycardia ablations. The death rate for atrial fibrillation ablations has been estimated at 0.2 percent (Cappato et al. 2009). The death rate for ventricular tachycardia ablations has been estimated at 1 to 2 percent (Peichl et al. 2014). A recent study (Santangeli et al. 2017) reported a 5 percent rate of death within one month of VT ablations with more than half of the deaths occurring while the patients were still hospitalized. The most common cause of in-hospital death is myocardial infarction (heart attack); less common causes include pulmonary embolism, stroke, heart failure, and sepsis.

Length of hospital stay. Most patients who undergo EP studies and ablation go home the next day; many patients who undergo EP studies and ablations for atrial fibrillation or ventricular tachycardia will stay more than one night in the hospital. I have found that older patients may have longer lengths of stay in the hospital. Patients who undergo EP studies and ablations but were hospitalized for other reasons (e.g., they were not electively admitted to the hospital for their EP study) tend to have longer lengths of stay in the hospital.

Hospital readmission. Many patients undergoing EP studies have heart failure, and these patients have higher readmission rates than patients without heart failure. Furthermore, patients who undergo EP studies and ablations but were hospitalized for other reasons (e.g., they were not electively admitted to the hospital for their EP study) tend to have longer lengths of stay in the hospital *and* higher rates of hospital readmission.

There are many factors that can increase the likelihood of readmission to the hospital after an EP study. Increased age and increased ablation complexity (e.g., ablations that only involve the right side of the heart are less complex than ablations that require transseptal punctures to gain access to the left side of the heart) may increase readmission rate. Other factors that can increase risk of readmission include abnormal kidney function, emergency situation/presentation, ejection fraction, female gender, and small stature (weight less than one hundred pounds). Reasons for readmission are quite varied, but many result from the aforementioned complications in addition to heart failure, pneumonia, or strokes. Many patients who require EP studies are greater than sixty-five years of age and often have other medical conditions that may be exacerbated by any surgical procedure.

Strokes. Strokes (also called *transient ischemic attacks* [TIAs]) may occur immediately postoperatively or can occur several weeks after implantation. Strokes generally occur in less than 1 percent of patients but have been seen in up to 1 percent of patients undergoing atrial fibrillation ablations (Cappato et al. 2009). I have most commonly seen strokes in patients who had anticoagulation (warfarin or Coumadin) held temporarily for the surgery; the strokes occur during the time the anticoagulation was held until the patient has been effectively re-anticoagulated after the surgery. There are data to suggest that EP procedures can be safely performed without stopping warfarin, which may lead to fewer complications (Ahmed et al. 2010). It is important to discuss management of anticoagulants with the implanting physician prior to surgery.

Special EP studies and ablations that may have higher rates of complications and lower success rates. *Ablations for atrial fibrillation* are viewed as higher-risk ablations for several reasons. First, ablations for atrial fibrillation involve accessing the left atrium of the heart and require one (or more) trans-septal punctures. These punctures are technically demanding and may result in inadvertent damage to your heart and vascular system. Furthermore, most patients are given strong blood thinners before, during, and after the ablation, thus exacerbating any procedural risks. Second, atrial fibrillation ablations can require tens (or hundreds) of ablation lesions; there is risk any time a burn (ablation) is delivered to the heart. Finally, the success rate for atrial fibrillation ablation ranges from 60 to 80 percent for a single procedure, and over 50 percent of patients may require more than one procedure to control symptoms from atrial fibrillation (Wynn et al. 2016). Of patients undergoing an ablation for atrial fibrillation, approximately 15 percent of patients may require a repeat ablation within one year of the initial procedure, and approximately 30 percent of these patients will require a repeat ablation within three years of the initial procedure. The death rate for atrial fibrillation ablations has been estimated at 0.2 percent (Cappato et al. 2009).

Ablations for ventricular tachycardia (VT) are also viewed as higher-risk ablations. As with atrial fibrillation ablations, VT ablations often require transseptal punctures to gain access to the left ventricle, which is a common site of origin for VT. Patients undergoing these ablations may also be on anticoagulation and need large numbers of ablations (burns). More importantly, the vast majority of patients with VT also have underlying severe coronary-artery blockages as well as heart failure; these patients are at higher risk of procedural heart attacks and death. Most patients who have VT from coronary-artery blockages will have several different types of VT, with each requiring its own special type of ablation (usually completed during the same procedure). It is estimated that 60 percent of patients who undergo ablations for VT will have recurrent VT within six months of the EP study! The death rate for ventricular tachycardia ablations has been estimated at 1 to 2 percent (Peichl et al. 2014). A recent study (Santangeli et al. 2017) reported a 5 percent rate of death within one month of VT ablations with more than half of the deaths occurring while the patients were still hospitalized.

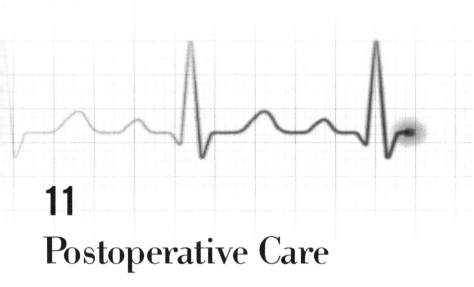

11
Postoperative Care

Each electrophysiologist and practice will have slightly different postoperative-care instructions, and it is important to check with your doctor regarding special instructions after electrophysiology (EP) studies with or without ablations. The limitations/restrictions I generally recommend to patients following EP studies are summarized in this chapter. However, my postoperative care sometimes varies, depending on a particular patient's medical problems. You should confirm activity limitations/restrictions with your doctor after the procedure.

Care of the vascular access sites (showering/bathing). Proper healing of the incision is critical to avoid infections of the vascular access sites after the EP study. For this reason, I recommend no tub baths or showers for seven days after the EP study—the average duration of restriction ranges from two to fourteen days. The patient should not get water, soap, ointments, or salves on or near the access sites during this time (unless instructed otherwise by the physician). Proper postoperative wound care is critical for a successful EP study even if the arrhythmia was ablated. Once the access sites have healed during this initial period, the patient can begin showering, and any superficial bandages will begin to fall off on their own.

It is normal for the access sites to be sore for several days to weeks after the EP study. There will be mild tenderness at the sites that should improve on a daily basis. If the pain is getting worse or the site gets redder or more swollen or feels hot, the patient should call the operating physician. The vast majority of my patients require only nonnarcotic pain relief (e.g., Advil or Tylenol) after the procedure; a few patients may require narcotic pain relief.

The site itself may look slightly red for the first several days, but it should get less and less red each day. If there is any increasing redness, warmth, or swelling, the operating physician should be notified. You may see some dried blood over the access site, and this can be normal; if bleeding persists or if the site continues to ooze or leak fluid, the operating physician should be notified. The vascular access sites may have some small areas (less than the size of a pea) of firmness and mild soft-tissue swelling in a site that is healing normally. There should be no significant tension at the access site; the groin site should not look like it is being "stretched" because of swelling underneath. A groin hematoma is an abnormal collection of blood overlying the site where the blood vessel was entered but underneath the incision; it looks like swelling. As long as there is no abnormal redness or tenderness, a small hematoma will usually heal slowly over the next several days to weeks. Again, any concern about the incision healing should be relayed to your doctor.

Symptoms that should be reported immediately to a physician include the following:

- fevers or chills
- incisional redness, warmth, tenderness, or swelling
- drainage or bleeding from the incision site
- chest pain, shortness of breath, or difficult breathing
- hiccups or abnormal "twitching" of muscles of the chest wall or rib cage
- swelling in the arms, wrists, legs, or ankles

- fainting (syncope), lightheadedness, or dizziness
- palpitations or fast, racing heartbeat
- severe weakness or fatigue
- any dramatic change or development of symptoms immediately following an EP study

Activity limitations. Patients should not do any vigorous exertion or lift more than five pounds for one week after the EP study. This activity limitation is more to allow the vascular access sites to heal rather than anything related to your heart. Clearly, contact sports and vigorous activity should be avoided during the first four weeks. You should ask your doctor about participating in any activity that may involve excessive jarring or trauma.

Driving. I generally recommend that patients not drive until the first follow-up appointment, which is normally ten to fourteen days after the EP study. This allows me to make sure the vascular access sites are healing properly and the patient has recovered appropriately. Obviously, patients who experienced any alterations in consciousness (fainting) prior to receiving the EP study should not drive until their physicians deem it safe to do so. Each state is different; Pennsylvania law, for example, suggests that patients may drive after six months if the reason for their fainting (syncope) can be fully explained and they have no further episodes of syncope during this time. It is recommended that the patient not drive for twelve months from the last episode of fainting if no cause is identified. Please check with your doctor before you resume driving.

The first follow-up appointment after the EP study. A follow-up visit is usually arranged for one to two weeks after the EP study. I have the patient return for a visit to assess the vascular access sites, symptoms, and medication tolerance and continue the education process. After this initial visit, the patient will be scheduled for in-office evaluation and ongoing education at a frequency appropriate for the patient's particular condition. Each physician offers different follow-up options.

Lifestyle considerations. One major concern for many arrhythmia patients is that symptoms will dramatically affect their lifestyles. Once temporary activity limitations are lifted (generally at two to four weeks), there are very few changes that need to be made. An important consideration for any arrhythmia patient is to plan for an exacerbation of arrhythmia issues when there is increased stress, decreased sleep, or use of caffeine, alcohol, or nicotine. I recommend that patients research hospitals and doctors in areas they will be visiting while traveling in case of emergency. Furthermore, it is important to ask your care provider if there are any medications that can be adjusted if there is an arrhythmia exacerbation while on vacation; this could be as simple as an extra or increased dose of beta-blockers or calcium-channel blockers.

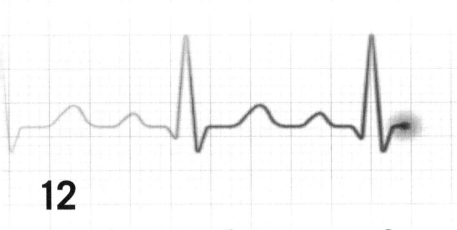

12

Psychosocial Impact of Arrhythmias

We have talked about the different types of arrhythmias and treatment options, but it is important to recognize that heart-rhythm abnormalities could cause or worsen emotional distress and have other psychosocial impacts.

Adjustment to life after being diagnosed with heart-rhythm abnormalities. One of the most important aspects of a patient's life after being diagnosed with an arrhythmia is understanding the risks (if any) of the particular type of arrhythmia. One can minimize this by saying, "You have an arrhythmia, and you have to get used to it!" Unfortunately, it is not this simple. Many arrhythmias—such as atrioventricular nodal reentrant tachycardia (AVNRT), atrial tachy-cardia, premature atrial contractions (PACs), and pre-mature ventricular contractions (PVCs)—are not life threatening, and I try to stress the benign (although annoying, from a symptomatic standpoint) nature of these heart-rhythm abnormalities; in patients with significant symptoms, these can be treated with medications and/or EP studies with ablations. Atrial fibrillation can be treated with blood thinners to min-imize possibly life-threatening strokes as well as anti-arrhythmics and/or ablations to decrease symptoms. Similarly, ventricular tachycardia can be treated with antiarrhythmics and/or ablations to decrease symp-toms.

Patients have accepted their arrhythmias when they understand their risks and treatment options and that quality of life can be restored in many (if not all) patients. Not only can emotional stress cause cardiac events, but there is some evidence that certain per-sonality traits can affect the long-term prognosis of heart-rhythm patients. Warning signs of patients who may have difficulty adjusting to their arrhythmias (and possibly have more heart-rhythm abnormalities) include patients with high levels of prediagnosis con-cerns as well as individuals who experience exces-sive worrying, depression, negativity, and anxiety (Pedersen et al. 2010).

Quality of life in heart-rhythm patients. *Quality of life* refers to the general well-being of a patient. Most heart-rhythm trials evaluated the burden of arrhythmias but did not particularly study the effects of these heart-rhythm problems on a patient's general well-being. Atrial fibrillation is the most common heart-rhythm disorder resulting in hospitalization. This arrhythmia (and most other supraventricular arrhythmias) is rarely life threatening, but it can cause significant distress and result in a major reduction in a patient's quality of life. Our current focus of managing these arrhythmias aims to reduce symptoms and prevent medical complications. The patient's psychological well-being is an important consideration of care providers.

How do arrhythmias affect you and your family? Not only can patients with arrhythmias experience depression or anxiety, but their life partners and family members may also experience psychological issues surrounding heart-rhythm management. This is often a two-way street. I think the most important aspect of dealing with heart-rhythm abnormalities is understanding the patient's condition. Clearly, this book is an important resource in helping patients to understand arrhythmias. Additionally, the significant other can accompany the patient to the office visits. This serves to inform the significant other about the disease process and also helps the patient to have another set of "ears" listening to the doctor's explanation and treatment recommendations. Lifestyle changes such as diet and exercise not only affect the patient but the significant other as well; when family and friends participate in these lifestyle changes, it often leads to a greater treatment success for the patient. Finally, depression can be an issue for cardiac patients. If the patient (or family member) exhibits signs or symptoms of depression (e.g., anger, withdrawal, difficulty sleeping, sadness), it is important to talk about it together. If symptoms are very concerning, it is important to talk to your doctors and other health-care providers.

Arrhythmias in children and young adults. It is important to convey to patients that arrhythmias can be troublesome, but most patients will live long and healthy lives. The patient will benefit from a "strong community of family or friends" (Dimsdale et al. 2012). Family and friends should have a keen eye for any signs of anxiety or depression and not hesitate to seek out help if they are worried about the patient. As the children grow older, they will seek out more independence and need more information about and control over their medical conditions. Family and friends should encourage the patient to participate in managing his or her own health (Dimsdale et al. 2012). Along the way, it is necessary to educate important adults in the child's life (e.g., teachers, coaches, and family friends) about the particular heart-rhythm abnormality and the child's health condition.

Can you have palpitations without arrhythmias?
Yes. I see many patients who have symptoms of palpitations with clear demonstration that there is no associated arrhythmia. After a thorough evaluation demonstrating no obvious heart abnormality, the most important thing we can offer the patient is reassurance that there is no obvious heart-rhythm abnormality. Conversely, I also have seen patients with over thirty years of symptoms of palpitations (and multiple evaluations by physicians), and we were finally able to find an arrhythmia! During those thirty years, we were just never able to document the occurrence of an arrhythmia. Some of these patients had symptoms that are not associated with arrhythmia, but ultimately, we were able to diagnose their arrhythmia. Be patient with your care provider, but always consider a second opinion as an option.

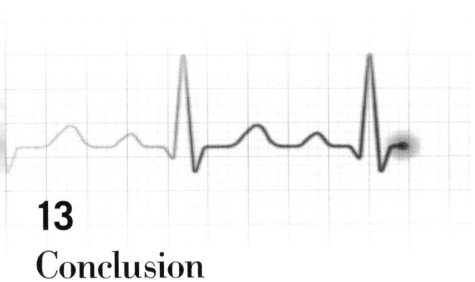

13
Conclusion

Millions of people have palpitations and arrhythmias, and as the population ages, more and more people will be living with advanced heart disease and battling heart-rhythm abnormalities. Hopefully, this comprehensive guide will provide patients and their families with a full explanation of the "what, why, and how" of heart-rhythm abnormalities.

This book provides an in-depth study of heart-rhythm abnormalities from initial patient evaluation through medical management and possible EP studies with ablations as well as the issues that may arise during long-term follow-up. I welcome the incorporation of this book into a typical plan of care for patients with heart-rhythm abnormalities, beginning with the initial discussions in the primary-care provider's office to serving as a long-term reference for patients who are undergoing treatment for arrhythmias. Indeed, I have found it to be a very useful component of the informed-consent process of my patients during the treatment of heart-rhythm issues.

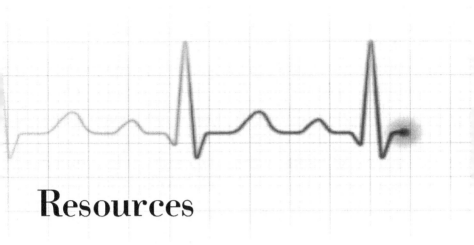

Resources

Heart.org: This is the website for the American Heart Association. You will find exhaustive resources for physicians and patients about cardiovascular disease and stroke. The organization Fellows of the American Heart Association (denoted by FAHA after a doctor's name) recognizes a particular physician's scientific and professional accomplishments, volunteer leadership, and service dedicated to cardiovascular medicine.

Cardiosmart.org: This is the website for the American College of Cardiology. There is extensive information about cardiology for the patient and provider. Fellows of the American College of Cardiology (denoted by FACC after their names) are selected based on their outstanding credentials, achievements, and community contributions to promote excellence in cardiovascular care.

Hrsonline.org: The Heart Rhythm Society (HRS) is a leading resource on cardiac pacing, defibrillators, and electrophysiology. This specialty organization represents medical, allied health, and science professionals, from more than seventy countries, who specialize in heart-rhythm disorders. HRS delivers programs and services to its membership. Fellows of the Heart Rhythm Society (denoted by FHRS after their names) have advanced training and certifications and have demonstrated a commitment to the research and treatment of heart-rhythm disorders.

Heart-rhythm-center.com: This is my discussion forum for biotechnology, pacemakers, defibrillators, and electrophysiology studies, including ablation. Patients and physicians can learn about and comment on a host of topics related to heart rhythms.

Device-manufacturer websites: The following is a list of the manufacturers of the most common implanted pacemaker and defibrillators and their websites. These websites often have patient and physician educational resources that are very informative:

1. Biotronik: www.biotronik.com

2. Boston Scientific Corporation: www.boston-scientific.com

3. Medtronic, Inc.: www.medtronic.com

4. Soren Group USA, Inc.: www.soren.com

5. St. Jude Medical, Inc.: www.sjm.com

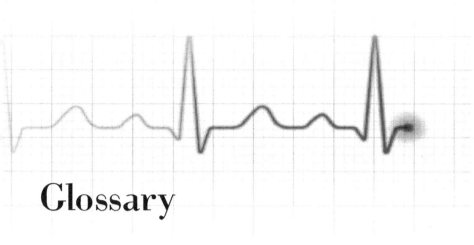

Glossary

Ablation: Catheter-based electrical heating (or super cooling, called cryoablation) of tissue that is used to treat arrhythmias in the electrophysiology laboratory.

Advisory: A warning issued to alert patients and care providers that a pacemaker or defibrillator or leads may be at risk for malfunction.

Amplitude: The level of voltage the heart generates or that a defibrillator lead delivers to the heart for pacing.

Anaphylaxis: Severe allergic reaction.

Anticoagulation: Thinning of the blood of a patient who may be on aspirin, warfarin, or heparin-based products.

Antitachycardia pacing (ATP): Rapid pacing delivered by a defibrillator or during an electrophysiology study to painlessly terminate an arrhythmia.

Aorta: The large vessel leaving the heart that carries blood to the rest of the body.

Aortic valve: The valve that blood crosses when it is pumped out of the heart and into the aorta.

Arrhythmia: A disruption of the orderly progression of SA-node activation through the AV node and the right and left ventricle. This abnormal heart rhythm may be too slow or too fast.

Arrhythmogenic: Characteristic of a medication, condition, or situation that can cause an abnormal heart rhythm.

Asymptomatic: Displaying a lack of symptoms.

Atelectasis: Minor collapse of lung airways that is common after surgeries and may cause fever or difficulty breathing.

Atrioventricular (AV) block: Electrical-conduction block between the top heart chambers (atrium) and the bottom heart chambers (ventricles). Pacemaker support may be necessary when you have an AV block.

Atrioventricular (AV) node: Specialized region of tissue that conducts electrical impulses from the top heart chambers (atrium) to the bottom heart chambers (ventricles).

Atrioventricular nodal reentrant tachycardia (AVNRT): This is a type of supraventricular tachycardia (SVT) that can cause palpitations and results from dual AV-node physiology.

Atrioventricular reentrant tachycardia (AVRT): This is a type of supraventricular tachycardia (SVT) that results from an extra (abnormal) electrical connection from the atria to the ventricles.

Atrium: Either of the top chambers of the heart that pumps the blood to the ventricles (plural, atria).

Axillary vein: The main vein that drains the arm; when the axillary vein enters the rib cage, it forms the subclavian vein.

Basilic vein: This vein drains blood from the arm and joins with the cephalic vein to form the axillary vein.

Bifascicular block: Electrical-system block below the atrioventricular node in the right and left bundle branches.

Biventricular: Refers to both the left and right ventricles and is generally used to describe a pacemaker or defibrillator that resynchronizes the left and right ventricles in patients with or at risk for heart failure.

Bradycardia: An abnormally slow heart rate of less than sixty beats per minute.

Brugada syndrome: A heart-rhythm disorder associated with electrocardiogram abnormalities that can cause sudden death.

Bundle branch: The left and right bundle branches are the major branches of the conduction system that provide electrical activation for the left and right ventricles; the left bundle branch has two major subdivisions called the left-anterior and left-posterior fascicles.

Capture: Term describing when an electrical pacing signal (voltage and current) causes atrial or ventricular tissue to contract (depolarize).

Cardiac-resynchronization therapy (CRT): A technique that uses an extra lead in the left ventricle so that the right and left ventricles pump at the same time.

Cardioinhibitory response: A decrease in heart rate and blood pumping that can cause a loss of consciousness.

Cardiologist: Internal medicine doctor whose training involves four years of undergraduate college, four years of medical school, three years of internal medicine residency, and three years of cardiology fellowship.

Cardiomyopathy: A disease process that can cause a loss of heart-muscle pumping ability and lead to heart failure.

Cardioversion: A procedure using electricity or medicines to convert an abnormally fast heart rhythm to a normal rhythm.

Catecholaminergic polymorphic ventricular tachycardia: A rare condition that may cause sudden death during stress or physical exertion.

Catheter: A small tube that can be inserted in the heart via a peripheral blood vessel in the arm or leg.

Catheterization: The process by which catheters are placed into the heart's chambers or coronary arteries.

Cephalic vein: A large vein that is often seen in the upper arm over the bicep muscle and joins with the basilica vein to form the axillary vein; this vein runs in the groove between the shoulder and chest muscles (called the deltopectoral groove).

Chronotropic incompetence: An inability to increase heart rate during exercise or exertion.

Clavicle: The medical name for the collarbone; pacemakers and defibrillators are generally implanted two finger breadths below the clavicle.

Complete heart block: A complete lack of electrical communication between the atrium and ventricles that often requires pacing when it is irreversible.

Congenital: Any abnormal heart condition a person is born with.

Congestive heart failure: The heart's inability to pump enough blood to the rest of the body.

Contraindication: Medical reason that prevents a patient from having a certain medication or procedure.

Contrast: Clear liquid that is used to highlight blood vessels and heart structure during some invasive procedures.

Contrast-induced nephropathy (CIN): Kidney damage that is caused by intravenous dye (called contrast) given during device implantation.

Coronary artery: Blood vessel that runs on the outside of the heart (epicardium) and provides oxygenated blood to the heart muscle; the left main coronary artery branches into the left-anterior descending and left circumflex: these generally supply blood to the left side of the heart (left atrium and ventricle); the right coronary artery generally supplies blood to the right side of the heart (right atrium and ventricle).

Coronary sinus: This is the major vein that drains blood from the heart muscle and directs it back toward the right atrium so that blood can be reoxygenated in the lungs; the coronary sinus allows placement of pacemaker leads that are used to pace the left ventricle to enable resynchronization therapy.

Creatinine: A blood laboratory test that indicates kidney function.

Cryoablation: Catheter-based super cooling of tissue that is used to treat arrhythmias in the electrophysiology laboratory.

Cryptogenic stroke: A "brain attack" without an obvious cause.

Current: Flow of electric charge through pacemaker or defibrillator leads.

Defibrillator: Device that is used to terminate life-threatening arrhythmias. A defibrillator can be fully implantable or applied externally by paramedics.

Diaphragm: Muscle responsible for causing the lungs to expand during breathing; the phrenic nerve can be inadvertently paced, causing a "hiccup" sensation (called diaphragmatic stimulation).

Diastolic: Refers to the time of minimum blood pressure during relaxation of the heart between beats. Diastolic heart failure is when your heart does not relax effectively between heartbeats.

Dislodgement: Term describing when a lead moves out of position after a pacemaker or defibrillator implantation, which may cause the lead to malfunction.

Dissection: Tear in a blood vessel that may require treatment.

Dyssynchrony: Failure of the right and left ventricles of the heart to contract at the same time; often present in heart-failure patients.

Echocardiogram: Special type of ultrasound (or sonogram) that uses sound waves to assess the structure and function of the heart.

Edema: Swelling from excess fluid in your body's tissues. Edema may be found in your lungs, abdomen, hands or legs.

Effusion: Collection of blood or fluid around the heart or lungs.

Ejection fraction (EF): Amount of blood that is pumped by the heart during a normal heartbeat; a normal EF is between 55 and 70 percent.

Elective replacement indicator (ERI): Alert on a defibrillator or pacemaker that signals it is necessary for the battery to be replaced; generally, devices can function for several weeks to months once they reach ERI.

Electrocardiogram (ECG or EKG): Apparatus that records the electrical activity of the heart, via electrodes that are placed on a patient's chest; the ECG is an important tool that cardiologists use to evaluate for disease.

Electrolytes: These are elements/minerals that are found in the blood and are important for normal heart function; they can cause heart-rhythm abnormalities and are measured as part of routine laboratory test during outpatient evaluations or in preparation for procedures.

Electrophysiologist: Subspecialized cardiologist who has extra training and expertise to perform heart-rhythm evaluations, EP studies/ablations, and electrophysiology-device implants, such as pacemakers and defibrillators.

Electrophysiology (EP): Study of heart-rhythm disorders.

Electrophysiology (EP) study: Term describing a procedure in which a specialized cardiologist (cardiac electrophysiologist) places catheters inside the heart to record and assess the heart's electrical function.

End of life (EOL): Alert on a pacemaker or defibrillator that signifies that the battery is very close to empty; at EOL, the pacemaker or defibrillator can behave erratically and even fail.

Endocardium: The inside lining of the heart muscle that is in direct contact with the blood.

Epicardium: The outside lining of the heart that is in contact with the pericardium; coronary arteries are found here.

Erosion: Thinning of the skin over a pacemaker or defibrillator that can lead to infection.

Fascicle: Branches of the heart's conduction system that are called the left-anterior and posterior fascicles.

Fibrillation: Very fast beating of the heart that can be seen in the atrium (not generally fatal) or ventricle (often fatal).

Fistula: Abnormal connection between arteries and veins that can be caused by vascular access during heart procedures.

Fixation: Term describing how leads are attached to the heart during pacemaker or defibrillator implantations; active fixation involves a small helix that is screwed into the heart; passive fixation involves small, soft fingers that are wedged into the lining of the heart to stay attached (like the barbs of a fishhook).

Fluoroscopy: Special type of imaging that allows the doctor to perform x-rays while the patient or the heart is moving. Fluoroscopy is used during procedures to guide catheters or place pacemaker/defibrillator leads into the heart.

Header: Block at the top of a pacemaker or defibrillator where the leads are connected.

Heart attack: Sudden blockage of a coronary artery, often referred to as a myocardial infarction (MI) by care providers.

Hematoma: Abnormal collection of blood that can cause swelling of a vascular access site or the implant site for a pacemaker or defibrillator.

Hemodynamics: Study of blood flow and the body's circulation; some pacemakers have features that can detect hemodynamic indicators such as fluid retention, activity, and respiratory motion.

Hemothorax: Abnormal collection of blood around the lungs in the chest that can result from any procedure involving your heart; it can be detected by an echocardiogram or chest x-ray.

High-frequency jet ventilation: A special form of ventilation that is used to minimize respiratory motion during a surgical procedure.

His-Purkinje: Fibers of the conduction system in the bottom heart chambers (ventricles).

Hydration: Overall water content of a patient and/or the process of replacing or adding to the water content of a patient.

Hypertension: Elevated blood pressure.

Hyperthyroid: Abnormally elevated thyroid function.

Hypertrophic cardiomyopathy: Type of heart disease that causes a much-thickened heart muscle and can cause sudden death (particularly in young athletes).

Hypotension: Low blood pressure.

Hypothyroid: Abnormally decreased thyroid function.

Impedance: Measure of the opposition in current that is present in a pacemaker or defibrillator lead.

Inappropriate shock or therapy: Occurrence of unnecessary (and potentially harmful) shocks or pacing when the defibrillator erroneously senses (is "fooled into" thinking) that a patient is having a life-threatening arrhythmia.

Indication: Medical reason for a particular procedure, therapy, or medication.

Infarction: Dead heart-muscle cells caused by a heart attack; another name for a heart attack is myocardial infarction (MI).

Interrogation: Process of checking the function of an implanted pacemaker or defibrillator; it can be done at the bedside, in the office, or remotely while the patient is at home.

Ischemic cardiomyopathy: Heart failure caused by blocked coronary arteries.

Long-QT syndrome: Disease of heart-muscle cells that leads to electrocardiogram abnormalities and is a cause of sudden, unexpected death.

Mitral valve: One-way valve that blood crosses when traveling from the left atrium to the left ventricle.

Mixed cardiomyopathy: Heart failure that has more than one cause, such as heart failure due to a combination of coronary-artery blockages and a leaking valve.

Morbidity: Risk of complications, injuries, or symptoms from a device implantation.

Mortality: Risk of death from a device implantation.

Myocardium: Heart muscle. Myocardial cells make up the myocardium.

Myopotential: Electrical potential that is created by muscle outside the heart—such as the diaphragm—that can be sensed by a pacemaker or defibrillator and cause an inappropriate shock or pause in pacing.

Nephropathy: Damage to the kidneys.

Nonischemic cardiomyopathy: Heart failure in a patient with no significant coronary-artery blockages.

Occlusion: Stoppage of blood flow through a blood vessel. If a *stenosis* is severe enough, the blood vessel can close off and result in occlusion.

Oversensing: Abnormal detection of signals by a pacemaker or defibrillator that can cause malfunction.

P wave: Component of the electrocardiogram that corresponds to the activation and contraction of the top heart chambers (right and left atria).

Pacemaker: Device that is used to maintain a normal heart rate.

Perforation: Hole in one of the heart's chambers, arteries, or veins.

Pericardiocentesis: Process of removing an abnormal collection of blood (pericardial effusion) surrounding the heart.

Pericardium: Thin sac that lines the outside of the heart; blood collecting between the outside of the heart and this lining is called a pericardial effusion.

Phantom shock: Pain of a defibrillator shock experienced by the patient when no shock was actually delivered by the device.

Phlebitis: Inflammation or irritation of a blood vessel.

Phrenic nerve: Nerve that controls the diaphragm.

Pleura: Thin linings that surround the lungs and other organs inside the chest.

Pneumothorax: Abnormal collection of air outside the lungs that can be seen after a pacemaker implantation.

Premature atrial contractions (PACs; also referred to as atrial premature contractions [APCs] and atrial premature depolarizations [APDs]): These are extra signals from the top chambers (atria) that can trigger an extra heartbeat that interrupts the regular rhythm. They are very common and generally harmless, although they may cause symptoms if they occur frequently.

Premature ventricular contractions (PVCs; also referred to as ventricular premature contractions [VPCs] and ventricular premature depolarizations [VPDs]): These are extra signals from the bottom chambers (ventricles) that can trigger an extra heartbeat that interrupts the regular rhythm. They are very common and generally harmless, although they may cause symptoms if they occur frequently.

Primary prevention: Prevention of the first occurrence of a fatal arrhythmia in a patient with risk factors.

Programmer: Desktop computer that is used to interrogate a pacemaker or defibrillator to check function and program pacemaker features.

Prophylaxis: Medication used to prevent a reaction or infection.

Pulmonary valve: One-way valve that blood crosses when traveling from the right ventricle to the lungs.

Pulse width: Duration of a signal, in milliseconds, that is used to pace the heart.

QRS complex: Component of the electrocardiogram that corresponds to the activation and contraction of the bottom heart chambers (right and left ventricles).

Resynchronization: Pacing feature that restores the pumping action of the heart so that the right and left ventricles pump at the same time.

Secondary prevention: Prevention of another occurrence of a fatal arrhythmia in a patient who has had an initial event.

Shock plan: Action plan for what to do upon receiving a shock from an implanted defibrillator.

Shocks: Term describing the defibrillator's method to terminate arrhythmias by delivering bursts of high voltages to "reset" the heart and stop the harmful arrhythmias. They may be painful if the patient is conscious during shocks.

Short-QT syndrome: Heart-rhythm disorder associated with electrocardiogram abnormalities that can cause sudden death.

Sinoatrial (SA) node: Natural pacemaker of the heart located in the right atrium.

Sleep apnea: Sleep disorder that causes pauses in or abnormally slow breathing during sleep.

Stenosis: Blockage in a vein or artery. Device leads can cause the veins they are placed in to become stenosed.

Stethoscope: Tool used by care providers to listen to the heart.

Stroke: Stoppage of blood flow to a part of the brain; strokes are also called transient ischemic attacks (TIAs) or "brain attacks."

Subclavian vein: The vein located under the collar-bone that carries blood to the heart; it is used to place catheters into the heart or implant pacemaker or defibrillator leads.

Subcutaneous defibrillator: Special type of defibrillator that does not involve leads placed through the chest wall into the venous system. This is a type of defibrillator that does not offer routine pacing ability.

Sudden cardiac death: An unexpected death due to heart issues that occurs within one hour of symptom onset. A person can survive sudden cardiac death if resuscitation with a defibrillator is performed quickly.

Supraventricular tachycardia: An abnormally fast heart rhythm of greater than one hundred beats per minute that starts in the upper chambers of the heart (the right and left atria).

Synchrony: Simultaneous pumping of the right and left ventricles.

Syncope: Loss of consciousness; fainting.

Systolic: Refers to the time of maximum blood pressure during contraction of the heart. Systolic heart failure is when your heart cannot contract strongly enough.

T wave: Component of the electrocardiogram that corresponds to the relaxation and resetting of the bottom heart chambers (right and left ventricles).

Tachycardia: Abnormally fast heart rate above one hundred beats per minute.

Tachycardia-induced cardiomyopathy: Heart failure caused by an arrhythmia (such as atrial fibrillation) that causes the heart to beat very fast for sustained periods of time.

Tamponade: Dangerous pressure buildup outside the heart when blood collects between the outside of the heart (epicardium) and the sac that contains the heart (pericardium).

Therapies: Features that defibrillators use to terminate ventricular arrhythmias. Therapies include antitachy-cardia pacing and shocks.

Threshold: Energy (voltage and current) required to cause the heart to beat (this is called capture).

Thrombosis: Blood clot.

Tilt-table test: Method to evaluate causes of syncope that involves placing a patient on a table that tilts up to a steep angle and watching for changes in blood pressure and heart rate that cause symptoms.

Time-out: When the doctors, nurses, technologists, and all personnel who are participating in a surgery stop what they are doing (before the patient is sedated) and identify the patient, procedure being performed (including site of implant), technique to be used, and any other important patient information (such as drug allergies).

Transient ischemic attack (TIA): See *Stroke.*

Transvenous defibrillator: Most common type of defibrillator that uses leads placed through veins and attached to the heart.

Tricuspid valve: One-way valve that blood crosses when traveling from the right atrium to the right ventricle.

Twiddling: Manipulation of a pacemaker or defibrillator that may lead to malfunction.

Undersensing: Failure of a pacemaker or defibrillator to detect native heart signals that can lead to inappropriate pacing or failure to shock a potentially life-threatening arrhythmia.

Vagal maneuvers: Actions that stimulate the vagus nerve and slow the heart rate and include things like bearing down as if you were having a bowel movement, coughing vigorously, and placing your face in a bowl of ice water. These maneuvers cause your heart to slow conduction through the AV node and may terminate an arrhythmia.

Valvular cardiomyopathy: Heart failure caused by valve disease.

Vegetation: Collection of bacteria, forming a mass that adheres to the inside of your heart or pacemaker or defibrillator leads.

Vena cava: The inferior and superior vena cavae are the main vessels that return the body's blood to the right atrium.

Venography: X-ray of the veins taken after contrast is injected to assess if a pacemaker lead can be inserted.

Ventricle, left or right: Main pumping chambers that pump blood to the lungs and the rest of the body.

Ventricular fibrillation: Very fast beating of the bottom chambers of the heart (ventricles); is often fatal. Ventricular fibrillation is very different from atrial fibrillation.

Voltage: Electrical charge that can be measured or emitted by a pacemaker or defibrillator.

Wand: Small device placed on the chest over a pacemaker or defibrillator and connected by a wire to the programmer; the wand enables the pacemaker or defibrillator to communicate with the programmer.

X-ray: Special type of radiation used in medicine that is used to image bones and soft tissue.

Works Cited

Ahmed, I., E. Gertner, W. B. Nelson, C. M. House, R. Dahiya, C. P. Anderson, D. G. Benditt, and D. W. Zhu. 2010. "Continuing Warfarin Therapy Is Superior to Interrupting Warfarin with or without Bridging Anticoagulation Therapy in Patients Undergoing Pacemaker and Defibrillator Implantation." *Heart Rhythm* 7 (6): 745–49.

Avidan, M. S., E. Jacobsohn, D. Glick, B. A. Burnside, L. Zhang, A. Villafranca, L. Karl, S. Kamal, B. Torres, M. O'Connor, A. S. Evers, S. Gradwohl, N. Lin, B. J. Palanca, and George A. Mashour. 2011. "Prevention of Intraoperative Awareness in a High-Risk Surgical Population." *New England Journal of Medicine* 365: 591–600.

Brockow, K., C. Christiansen, G. Kanny, O. Clément, A. Barbaud, A. Bircher, P. Dewachter, J. L. Guéant, R. M. Rodriguez Guéant, C. Mouton-Faivre, J. Ring, A. Romano, J. Sainte-Laudy, P. Demoly, W. J. Pichler, ENDA, and the EAACI Interest Group on Drug Hypersensitivity. 2005. "Management of Hypersensitivity Reactions to Iodinated Contrast Media." *Allergy* 60: 150–58.

Cappato, R., H. Calkins, S. Chen, W. Davies, Y. Iesaka, J. Kalman, Y. Kim, G. Klein, A. Natale, D. Packer, and A. Skanes. 2009. "Prevalence and Causes of Fatal Outcome in Catheter Ablation of Atrial Fibrillation." *Journal of the American College of Cardiology* 53 (19): 1798–803.

Chen, S-A., C-E. Chiang, C-T. Tai, C. C. Cheng, C. W. Chio, S. H. Lee, K. C. Ueng, Z. C. Wen, M. S. Chang.1996. "Complications of Diagnostic Electrophysiologic Studies and Radiofrequency Catheter Ablation in Patients with Tachyarrhythmias: An Eight-Year Survey of 3,966 Consecutive Procedures in a Tertiary Referral Center." *American Journal of Cardiology* 77: 41–46.

Cheng, A., Y. Wang, J. P. Curtis, and P. D. Varosy. 2010. "Acute Lead Dislodgements and In-Hospital Mortality in Patients Enrolled in the National Cardiovascular Data Registry Implantable Cardioverter Defibrillator Registry." *Journal of the American College of Cardiology* 56: 1651–56.

Chow, G. V., J. E. Marine, and J. L. Fleg. 2012. "Epidemiology of Arrhythmias and Conduction Disorders in Older Adults." *Clinics in Geriatric Medicine* 28 (4): 539–553.

Curtis, J. P., J. J. Luebbert, Y. Wang, S. S. Rathore, J. Chen, P. A. Heidenreich, S. C. Hammill, R. I. Lampert, and H. M. Krumholz. 2009. "Association of Physician Certification and Outcomes among Patients Receiving an Implantable Cardioverter-Defibrillator." *The Journal of the American Medical Association* 301 (16): 1661–70.

DiBiase, L., S. Conti, P. Mohanty, R. Bai, J. Sanchez, D. Walton, A. John, P. Santangeli, C. S. Elayi, S. Beheiry, G. J. Gallinghouse, S. Mohanty, R. Horton, S. Bailey, J. D. Burkhardt, and A. Natale. 2011. "General Anesthesia Reduces the Prevalence of Pulmonary Vein Reconnection during Repeat Ablation When Compared with Conscious Sedation: Results from a Randomized Study." *Heart Rhythm* 8: 368–72.

Dimsdale, C., A. Dimsdale, J. Ford, J. B. Shea, and S. F. Sears. 2012. "My Child Needs or Has an Implantable Defibrillator: What Should I Do?" *Circulation* 126: e244–47.

Farling, P. A. 2000. "Thyroid Disease." *British Journal of Anaesthesia* 85 (1): 15–28.

Gaitan, B. D., T. L. Trentman, S. L. Fassett, J. T. Mueller, and G. T. Altemose. 2011. "Sedation and Analgesia in the Cardiac Electrophysiology Laboratory: A National Survey of Electrophysiologists Investigating the Who, How, and Why." *Journal of Cardiothoracic and Vascular Anesthesia* 25: 647–59.

Geyfman, V., R. H. Storm, S. C. Lico, and J. W. Oren, IV. 2007. "Cardiac Tamponade as Complication of Active-Fixation Atrial Lead Perforations: Proposed Mechanism and Management Algorithm." *Pacing and Clinical Electrophysiology* 30: 498–501.

Gopinathannair, R., S. P. Etheridge, F. E. Marchlinski, F. G. Spinale, D. Lakkireddy, and B. Olshansky. 2015. "Arrhythmia-Induced Cardiomyopathies: Mechanisms, Recognition, and Management." *Journal of the American College of Cardiology* 66 (15): 1714–28.

Hampton, J. R., M. J. F. Harrison, J. R. A. Mitchell, J. F. Prichard, and C. Seymour. 1975. "Relative Contributions of History-Taking, Physical Examination, and Laboratory Investigation to Diagnosis and Management of Medical Outpatients." *British Medical Journal* 2: 486–89.

Hautmann, H., F. Gamarra, M. Henke, S. Diehm, and R. M. Huber. 2000. "High-Frequency Jet Ventilation in Interventional Fiberoptic Bronchoscopy." *Anesthesia and Analgesia* 90:1436–40.

Hemmes, S. N. T., P. Severgnini, S. Jaber, J. Canet, H. Wrigge, M. Hiesmayr, E. M. Tschernko, M. W. Hollmann, J. M. Binnekade, G. Hedenstierna, C. Putensen, M. G. de Abreu, P. Pelosi, M. J. Schultz. 2011. "Rationale and Study Design of PROVHILO: A Worldwide Multicenter Randomized Controlled Trial on

Protective Ventilation during General Anesthesia for Open Abdominal Surgery." *Trials* 12: 111–121.

Hindricks, G. 1993. "The Multicentre European Radiofrequency Survey (MERFS): Complications of Radiofrequency Catheter Ablation of Arrhythmias." *European Heart Journal* 14: 1644–53.

Hunt, S. A., D. W. Baker, M. H. Chin, M. P. Cinquegrani, A. M. Feldman, G. S. Francis, T. G. Ganiats, S. Goldstein, G. Gregoratos, M. L. Jessup, R. J. Noble, M. Packer, M. A. Silver, L. W. Stevenson, R. J. Gibbons, E. M. Antman, J. S. Alpert, D. P. Faxon, V. F. A. K. Jacobs, L. F. Hiratzka, R. O. Russell, and S. C. Smith. 2001. "ACC/AHA Guidelines for the Evaluation and Management of Chronic Heart Failure in the Adult: Executive Summary: A Report of the American College of Cardiology/American Heart Association Task Force on Practice Guidelines (Committee to Revise the 1995 Guidelines for the Evaluation and Management of Heart Failure)." *Circulation* 104: 2996–3007.

Jaquet, Y., P. Monnier, G. Van Melle, P. Ravussin, D. R. Spahn, and M. Chollet-Rivier. 2006.

"Complications of Different Ventilation Strategies in Endoscopic Laryngeal Surgery." *Anesthesiology* 104: 52–59.

Lawrence, V. A., S. G. Hilsenbeck, C. D. Mulrow, R. Dhanda, J. Sapp, and C. P. Page. 1995. "Incidence and Hospital Stay for Cardiac and Pulmonary Complications after Abdominal Surgery." *Journal of General Internal Medicine* 10: 671–78.

Magnusson, L., and D. R. Spahn. 2003. "New Concepts of Atelectasis during General Anesthesia." *British Journal of Anaesthesia* 91 (1): 61–72.

Mahapatra, S., K. A. Bybee, T. J. Bunch, R. E. Espinosa, L. J. Sinak, M. D. McGoon, and D. L. Hayes. 2005. "Incidence and Predictors of Cardiac Perforation after Permanent Pacemaker Implantation." *Heart Rhythm* 2: 907–11.

Marcos, S. K., and H. S. Thomsen. 2001. "Prevention of General Reactions to Contrast Media: A Consensus Report and Guidelines." *European Radiology* 11 (9): 1720–28.

Murkin, J. M. 1982. "Anesthesia and Hypothyroidism: A Review of Thyroxine Physiology,

Pharmacology, and Anesthetic Implications." *Anesthesia and Analgesia* 61 (4): 371–83.

O'Hara, G. E., F. Philippon, J. Champagne, L. Blier, F. Molin, J-M. Côté, I. Nault, J-F. Sarrazin, and M. Gilbert. 2007. "Catheter Ablation for Cardiac Arrhythmias: A 14-Year Experience with 5330 Consecutive Patients at the Quebec Heart Institute, Laval Hospital." *Canadian Journal of Cardiology* 23(Suppl. B): 67B–70B.

Pedersen, S. S., K. C. van den Broek, R. A. M. Erdman, L. Jordaens, and D. A. M. J. Theuns. 2010. "Pre-implantation Implantable Cardioverter Defibrillator Concerns and Type D Personality Increase the Risk of Mortality in Patients with an Implantable Cardioverter Defibrillator." *Europace* 12: 1446–52.

Peichl, P., D. Wichterle, L. Pavlu, R. Cihak, B. Aldhoon, and J. Kautzner. 2014. "Complications of Catheter Ablation of Ventricular Tachycardia: A Single-Center Experience." *Circulation: Arrhythmia and Electrophysiology* 7(4): 684–90.

Probst, M. A., W. R. Mower, H. K. Kanzaria, J. R. Hoffman, E. F. Buch, and B. C. Sun. 2014.

"Analysis of Emergency Department Visits for Palpitations (from the National Hospital Ambulatory Medical Care Survey)." *American Journal of Cardiology* 113(10):1685–90.

Royal College of Radiologists. 2010. *Standards for Intravascular Contrast Administration to Adult Patients*. 2nd ed. London: Royal College of Radiologists.

Sebel, P. S., A. Bowdle, M. M. Ghoneim, I. J. Rampil, R. E. Padilla, T. J. Gan, K. B. Domino. 2004. "The Incidence of Awareness during Anesthesia: A Multicenter United States Study." *Anesthesia and Analgesia* 2004 99: 833–39.

Sohail, M. R., S. Hussain, K. Y. Le, C. Dib, C. M. Lohse, P. A. Friedman, D. L. Hayes, D. Z. Uslan, W. R. Wilson, J. M. Steckelberg, L. M. Baddour, and Mayo Cardiovascular Infections Study Group. 2011. "Risk Factors Associated with Early- versus Late-Onset Implantable Cardioverter-Defibrillator Infections." *Journal of Interventional Cardiac Electrophysiology* 31(2): 171–83.

Tramer, M. R., E. von Elm, P. Loubeyre, and C. Hauser. 2006. "Pharmacologic Prevention of

Serious Anaphylactic Reactions Due to Iodin-ated Contrast Material: Systematic Review." *The British Medical Journal* 333: 675–78.

Trcka, J., C. Schmidt, C. S. Seitz, E. B. Brocker, G. E. Gross, and A. Trautman. 2008. "Anaphylaxis to Iodinated Contrast Materials: Nonallergic Hypersensitivity or IgE-Mediated Allergy? *American Journal of Roentgenology* 190 (3): 666–70.

Trentman, T. L., S. L. Fassett, J. T. Mueller, and G. T. Altemose. 2009. "Airway Interventions in the Cardiac Electrophysiology Laboratory: A Ret-rospective Review." *Journal of Cardiothoracic and Vascular Anesthesia* 23: 841–45.

Tung, R., N. G. Boyle, and K. Shivkumar. 2010. "Catheter Ablation of Ventricular Tachycar-dia." *Circulation*, 122 (3): e389-e391.

Wang, N. C., J. L. Williams, S. K. Jain, and A. Shal-aby. 2009. "Post-Pacemaker Pulsations." *American Journal of Medicine* 122: 345–47.

Williams, J. L., D. Lugg, R. Gray, D. Hollis, M. Stoner, and R. Stevenson. 2010. "Patient Demograph-ics, Complications, and Hospital Utilization in 250 Consecutive Device Implants of a New Community Hospital Electrophysiology Program." *American Heart Hospital Journal* 8 (1): 33–39.

Williams, J. L., and R. T. Stevenson. 2012. "Complications of Pacemaker Implantation." In *Current Issues and Recent Advances in Pacemaker Therapy*, edited by Attila Roka. http://www.intechopen.com/books/current-issues-and-recent-advances-in-pacemaker-therapy/complications_of_pacemaker_implantation.

Williams, J. L., V. Valencia, D. Lugg, R. Gray, D. Hollis, J. W. Toth, R. Benson, M. DeFranceso-Loukas, R. T. Stevenson, and P. J. Teiken. 2011. "High-Frequency Jet Ventilation during Ablation of Supraventricular and Ventricular Arrhythmias: Efficacy, Patient Tolerance and Safety." *The Journal of Innovations in Cardiac Rhythm Management* 2: 1–7.

Wynn, G.J., M. El-Kadri, I. Haq, M. Das, S. Modi, R. Snowdon, M. Hall, J. Waktare, D.M. Todd, and D. Gupta. 2016. "Long-term outcomes after ablation of persistent atrial fibrillation: an observational study over 6 years."

Open Heart 3:e000394. doi: 10.1136/openhrt-2015-000394.

Zado, E. S., D. J. Callans, C. D. Gottlieb, S. P. Kutalek, S. L. Wilbur, F. L. Samuels, S. E. Hessen, C. M. Movsowitz, J. M. Fontaine, S. E. Kimmel, F. E. Marchlinski. 2000. "Efficacy and Safety of Catheter Ablation in Octogenarians." *Journal of the American College of Cardiology* 35(2): 458–62.

Further Reading

Alt, E., R. Volker, and H. Blomer. 1987. "Lead Fracture in Pacemaker Patients." *Thoracic Cardiovascular Surgery* 35: 101–4.

Alter P., S. Waldhans, E. Plachta, R. Moosdorf, and W. Grimm. 2005. "Complications of Implantable Cardioverter Defibrillator Therapy in 440 Consecutive Patients." *Pacing and Clinical Electrophysiology* 28: 926–32.

Bardy, G. H., K. L. Lee, D. B. Mark, J. E. Poole, D. L. Packer, R. Boineau, M. Domanski, C. Troutman, J. Anderson, G. Johnson, S. E. McNulty, N. Clapp-Channing, L. D. Davidson-Ray, E. S. Fraulo, D. P. Fishbein, R. M. Luceri, and J. H. Ip, for the Sudden Cardiac Death in Heart Failure Trial (SCD-HeFT) Investigators. 2005. "Amiodarone or an Implantable

Cardioverter-Defibrillator for Congestive Heart Failure." *The New England Journal of Medicine* 352 (3): 225–37.

Bayliss C. E., D. S. Beanlands, and R. J. Baird. 1968. "The Pacemaker-Twiddler's Syndrome: A New Complication of Implantable Transvenous Pacemakers." *Canadian Medical Association Journal* 99: 371–73.

Belott, P. "How to Access the Axillary Vein." 2006. *Heart Rhythm* 3 (3): 366–69.

Bohm, A., A. Pinter, and I. Preda. 2002. "Ventricular Tachycardia Induced by a Pacemaker Lead." *Acta Cardiologica* 57 (1): 23–24.

Bracke, F., A. Meijer, and B. Van Gelder. 2003. "Venous Occlusion of the Access Vein in Patients Referred for Lead Extraction: Influence of Patient and Lead Characteristics." *Pacing and Clinical Electrophysiology* 26: 1649–52.

Bristow, M. R., L. A. Saxon, J. Boehmer, S. Krueger, D. A. Kass, T. De Marco, P. Carson, L. DiCarlo, D. DeMets, B. G. White, D. W. DeVries, and A. M. Feldman, for the Comparison of

Medical Therapy, Pacing, and Defibrillation in Heart Failure (COMPANION) Investigators. 2004. "Cardiac-Resynchronization Therapy with or without an Implantable Defibrillator in Advanced Chronic Heart Failure." *The New England Journal of Medicine* 350 (21): 2140–50.

Burns J. L., E. R. Serber, S. Keim, and S. Sears. 2005. "Measuring Patient Acceptance of Implantable Cardiac Device Therapy: Initial Psychometric Investigation of the Florida Patient Acceptance Survey." *Journal of Cardiovascular Electrophysiology* 16 (4): 384–90.

Carlson, M. D., and B. L. Wilkoff. 2006. "Recommendation from the HRS Task Force on Device Performance Policies and Guidelines." *Heart Rhythm* 3: 1250–73.

Chadha T. S., and M. A. Cohn. 1983. "Noninvasive Treatment of Pneumothorax with Oxygen Inhalation." *Respiration* 44 (2): 147–52.

Cherubini, A., J. Oristrell, X. Pla, C. Ruggiero, R. Ferretti, G. Diestre, A. M. Clarfield, P. Crome, C. Hertogh, V. Lesauskaite, G. I. Prada, K. Szczerbinska, E. Topinkova, J. Sinclair-Cohen,

D. Edbrooke, and G. H. Mills. 2011. "The Persistent Exclusion of Older Patients from Ongoing Clinical Trials Regarding Heart Failure." *Archives of Internal Medicine* 171 (6): 550–56.

Crilley, J. G., B. Herd, C. S. Khurana, C. A. Appleby, M. A. de Belder, A. Davies, and J. A. Hall. 1997. "Permanent cardiac pacing in elderly patients with recurrent falls, dizziness and syncope, and a hypersensitive cardioinhibitory reflex." *Postgraduate Medical Journal* 73: 415–18.

Curtis, A. B., S. J. Worley, P. B. Adamson, E. S. Chung, I. Niazi, L. Sherfesee, T. Shinn, and M. Sutton, for the Biventricular versus Right Ventricular Pacing in Heart Failure Patients with Atrioventricular Block (BLOCK HF) Trial Investigators. 2013. "Biventricular Pacing for Atrioventricular Block and Systolic Dysfunction." *The New England Journal of Medicine* 368: 1585–93.

DaCosta, S. S., N. A. Scalabrini, A. Costa, J. G. Caldas, and F. M. Martinelli. 2002. "Incidence and Risk Factors of Upper Extremity Deep Vein Lesions after Permanent Transvenous

Pacemaker Implant: A 6-Month Follow-Up Prospective Study." *Pacing and Clinical Electrophysiology* 25: 1301–1306.

Datta, G., A. Sarkar, and A. Haque. 2011. "An Uncommon Ventricular Tachycardia Due to Inactive PPM Lead." *ISRN Cardiology 2011.* doi:10.5402/2011/232648.

D'Ivernois, C., J. Lesage, and P. Blanc. 2008. "Where Are Left Ventricular Leads Really Implanted? A Study of 90 Consecutive Patients." *Pacing and Clinical Electrophysiology* 31 (5): 554–59.

Ellenbogen, K. A., A. S. Hellkamp, B. L. Wilkoff, J. L. Camunas, L. C. Love, T. A. Hadjis, K. L. Lee, and G. A. Lamas. 2003. "Complications Arising after Implantation of DDD Pacemakers: The MOST Experience." *American Journal of Cardiology* 92: 740–41.

Ellenbogen, K. A., M. A. Wood, D. M. Gilligan, M. Zmijewski, D. Mans, and the CAPSURE Z Investigators. 1999. "Steroid Eluting High Impedance Pacing Leads Decrease Short and Long-Term Current Drain: Results from a Multicenter Clinical Trial." *Pacing and Clinical Electrophysiology* 22 (1): 39–48.

Ellery, S. M., and V. E. Paul. 2004. "Complications of Biventricular Pacing." *European Heart Journal Supplements* 6 (Su D): D117–21.

Epstein, A. E., J. P. DiMarco, K. A. Ellenbogen, N. A. Estes, III, R. A. Freedman, L. S. Gettes, A. M. Gillinov, G. Gregoratos, S. C. Hammill, D. L. Hayes, M. A. Hlatky, L. K. Newby, R. L. Page, M. H. Schoenfeld, M. J. Silka, L. W. Stevenson, M. O. Sweeney, S. C. Smith Jr., A. K. Jacobs, C. D. Adams, J. L. Anderson, C. E. Buller, M. A. Creager, S. M. Ettinger, D. P. Faxon, J. L. Halperin, L. F. Hiratzka, S. A. Hunt, H. M. Krumholz, F. G. Kushner, B. W. Lytle, R. A. Nishimura, J. P. Ornato, R. L. Page, B. Riegel, L. G. Tarkington, C. W. Yancy, American College of Cardiology/American Heart Association Task Force on Practice Guidelines (Writing Committee to Revise the ACC/AHA/NASPE 2002 Guideline Update for Implantation of Cardiac Pacemakers and Antiarrhythmia Devices), American Association for Thoracic Surgery, and Society of Thoracic Surgeons. 2008. "ACC/AHA/HRS 2008 Guidelines for Device-Based Therapy of Cardiac Rhythm Abnormalities: A Report of the American College of Cardiology/ American Heart Association Task Force on

Practice Guidelines (Writing Committee to Revise the ACC/AHA/NASPE 2002 Guideline Update for Implantation of Cardiac Pacemakers and Antiarrhythmia Devices)." *Journal of the American College of Cardiology* 51 (21): e1–62.

Ezekowitz, J. A., P. W. Armstrong, and F. A. McAlister. 2003. "Implantable Cardioverter Defibrillators in Primary and Secondary Prevention: A Systematic Review of Randomized, Controlled Trials." *Annals of Internal Medicine* 138 (6): 445–52.

Ezekowitz, J. A., B. H. Rowe, D. M. Dryden, N. Hooton, B. Vandermeer, C. Spooner, and F. A. McAlister. 2007. "Systematic Review: Implantable Cardioverter Defibrillators for Adults with Left Ventricular Systolic Dysfunction." *Annals of Internal Medicine* 147: 252–62.

Faber, T. S., R. Gradinger, S. Treusch, C. Morkel, J. Brachmann, C. Bode, and M. Zehender. 2007. "Incidence of Ventricular Tachyarrhythmias during Permanent Pacemaker Therapy in Low-Risk Patients: Results from the German Multicentre EVENTS Study." *European Heart Journal* 28 (18): 2238–42.

Fahraeus T., and C. J. Hoijer. 2003. "Early Pacemaker Twiddler Syndrome." *Europace* 5: 279–81.

Ferguson Jr., T. B., C. L. Ferguson, K. Crites, and P. Crimmins-Reda. 1996. "The Additional Hospital Costs Generated in the Management of Complications of Pacemaker and Defibrillator Implantations." *The Journal of Thoracic and Cardiovascular Surgery* 111: 742–52.

Fortescue, E. B., C. L. Berul, F. Cecchin, E. P. Walsh, J. K. Triedman, and M. E. Alexander. 2005. "Comparison of Modern Steroid-Eluting Epicardial and Thin Transvenous Pacemaker Leads in Pediatric and Congenital Heart Disease Patients." *Journal of Interventional Cardiac Electrophysiology* 14 (1): 27–36.

Freedman, A., M. T. Rothman, and J. W. Mason. 1982. "Recurrent Ventricular Tachycardia Induced by an Atrial Synchronous Ventricular-Inhibited Pacemaker." *Pacing and Clinical Electrophysiology* 5 (4): 490–94.

Fung, J. W., J. Y. Chan, R. Omar, A. Hussin, Q. Zhang, G. Yip, K. H. Lam, F. Fang, and C. M. Yu. 2007. "The Pacing to Avoid Cardiac Enlargement (PACE) Trial: Clinical Background, Rationale,

Design, and Implementation." *Journal of Cardiovascular Electrophysiology* 18: 735–39.

Fyke, III, F. E. 1993. "Infraclavicular Lead Failure: Tarnish on a Golden Route." *Pacing and Clinical Electrophysiology* 16: 373–76.

Germano, J. J., M. Reynolds, V. Essebag, and M. E. Josephson. 2006. "Frequency and Causes of Implantable Cardioverter-Defibrillator Therapies: Is Device Therapy Proarrhythmic?" *American Journal of Cardiology* 97: 1255–61.

Goldenberg, I, A. J. Moss, W. J. Hall, S. McNitt, W. Zareba, M. L. Andrews, and D. S. Cannom. 2006. "Causes and Consequences of Heart Failure after Prophylactic Implantation of a Defibrillator in the Multicenter Automatic Defibrillator Implantation Trial II." *Circulation* 113: 2810–16.

Gould, P. A. 2008. "Outcome of Advisory ICD Replacement: One Year Follow-Up." *Heart Rhythm* 5 (12): 1675–81.

Grammes, J. A., C. M. Schulze, M. Al-Bataineh, G. A. Yesenosky, C. S. Saari, M. J. Vrabel, J. Horrow, M. Chowdhury, J. M. Fontaine, and S.

P. Kutalek. 2010. "Percutaneous Pacemaker and Implantable Cardioverter-Defibrillator Lead Extraction in 100 Patients with Intracardiac Vegetations Defined by Transesophageal Echocardiogram." *Journal of the American College of Cardiology* 55 (9): 886–94.

Groeneveld, P. W., M. A. Matta, J. J. Suh, F. Yang, and J. A. Shea. 2007. "Quality of Life among Implantable Cardioverter-Defibrillator Recipients in the Primary Prevention Therapeutic Era." *Pacing and Clinical Electrophysiology* 30: 463–71.

Hargreaves, M. R., A. Doulalas, and O. J. M. Ormerod. 1995. "Early Complications Following Dual Chamber Pacemaker Implantation: 10-Year Experience of a Regional Pacing Centre." *European Journal of Cardiac Pacing and Electrophysiology* 5 (3): 133–38.

Hayes, D. L., and R. E. Vlietstra. 1993. "Pacemaker Malfunction." *Annals of Internal Medicine* 119 (8): 828–35.

Hirschl, D. A., V. R. Jain, H. Spindola-Franco, J. N. Gross, and L. B. Haramati. 2007. "Prevalence and Characterization of Asymptomatic

Pacemaker and ICD Lead Perforation on CT." *Pacing and Clinical Electrophysiology* 30: 28–32.

Iesaka, Y., T. Pinakatt, A. J. Gosselin, and J. W. Lister. 1982. "Bradycardia Dependent Ventricular Tachycardia Facilitated by Myopotential Inhibition of a VVI Pacemaker." *Pacing and Clinical Electrophysiology* 5 (1): 23–29.

Johansen, J. B., O. D. Jørgensen, M. Møller, P. Arnsbo, P. T. Mortensen, and J. C. Nielsen. 2011. "Infection after Pacemaker Implantation: Infection Rates and Risk Factors Associated with Infection in a Population-Based Cohort Study of 46,299 Consecutive Patients." *European Heart Journal* 32 (8): 991–98.

Jordaens, L., E. Robbens, E. Van Wassenhove, and D. L. Clement. 1989. "Incidence of Arrhythmias after Atrial or Dual-Chamber Pacemaker Implantation." *European Heart Journal* 10 (2): 102–7.

Kikkenborg Berg, S., P. Moons, A. D. Zwisler, P. Winkel, B. D. Pederson, P. Ulrich Pederson, and J. Hastrup Svendsen. 2013. "Phantom Shocks in Patients with Implantable Cardioverter

Defibrillator: Results from a Randomized Rehabilitation Trial (COPE-ICD)." *Europace* 15 (10): 1463–67.

Klug, D., M. Balde, D. Pavin, F. Hidden-Lucet, J. Clementy, N. Sadoul, J. L. Rey, G. Lande, A. Lazarus, J. Victor, C. Barnay, B. Grandbastien, S. Kacet, and PEOPLE Study Group. 2007. "Risk Factors Related to Infections of Implanted Pacemakers and Cardioverter-Defibrillators." *Circulation* 116: 1349–55.

Knight, B. P., A. Desai, J. Coman, M. Faddis, and P. Yong. 2004. "Long-Term Retention of Cardiac Resynchronization Therapy." *Journal of the American College of Cardiology* 44 (1): 72–77.

Korte, T., H. Koditz, T. Paul, and J. Tebbenjohanns. 2004. "High Incidence of Appropriate and Inappropriate ICD Therapies in Children and Adolescents with Implantable Cardioverter Defibrillator." *Pacing and Clinical Electrophysiology* 27 (7): 924–32.

Kulvatunyou, N., A. Vijayasekaran, A. Hansen, J. L. Wynne, T. O'Keeffe, R. S. Friese, B. Joseph, A. Tang, and P. Rhee. 2011. "Two-Year

Experience of Using Pigtail Catheters to Treat Traumatic Pneumothorax: A Changing Trend." *Journal of Trauma* 71 (5): 1104–7.

Lee, D. S., A. D. Krahn, J. S. Healey, D. Birnie, E. Crystal, P. Dorian, C. S. Simpson, Y. Khaykin, D. Cameron, A. Janmohamed, R. Yee, P. C. Austin, Z. Chen, J. Hardy, and J. V. Tu. 2010. "Evaluation of Early Complications Related to De Novo Cardioverter Implantation." *Journal of the American College of Cardiology* 55 (8): 774–82.

Lauer, M. S., G. S. Francis, P. M. Okin, F. J. Pashkow, C. F. Snader, and T. H. Marwick. 1999. "Impaired Chronotropic Response to Exercise Stress Testing as a Predictor of Mortality." *Journal of the American Medical Association* 281: 524–29.

Lemon J., S. Edelman, and A. Kirkness. 2004. "Avoidance Behaviors in Patients with Implantable Cardioverter Defibrillators." *Heart and Lung* 33 (3): 176–82.

Leon, A. R., W. T. Abraham, A. B. Curtis, J. P. Daubert, W. G. Fisher, J. Gurley, D. L. Hayes, R. Lieberman, S. Petersen-Stejskal, K. Wheelan, and

MIRACLE Study Program. 2005. "Safety of Transvenous Cardiac Resynchronization System Implantation in Patients with Chronic Heart Failure: Combined Results of over 2000 Patients from a Multicenter Study Program." *Journal of the American College of Cardiology* 46 (12): 2348–56.

Li, W., B. Sarubbi, and J. Somerville. 2000. "Iatrogenic Ventricular Tachycardia from Endocardial Pacemaker Late after Repair of Tetralogy of Fallot." *Pacing and Clinical Electrophysiology* 23 (12): 2131–34.

Link, M. S., N. A. M. Estes, J. J. Griffin, P. J. Wang, J. D. Maloney, J. B. Kirchhoffer, G. F. Mitchell, J. Orav, L. Goldman, and G. A. Lamas. 1998. "Complications of Dual Chamber Pacemaker Implantation in the Elderly." *Journal of Interventional Cardiac Electrophysiology* 2: 175–79.

Lukl, J., V. Doupal, E. Sovová, and L. Lubena. 1999. "Incidence and Significance of Chronotropic Incompetence in Patients with Indications for Primary Pacemaker Implantation or Pacemaker Replacement." *Pacing and Clinical Electrophysiology* 22 (9): 1284–91.

Magney, J. E., D. M. Flynn, J. A. Parsons, D. H. Staplin, M. V. Chin-Purcell, S. Milstein, and D. W. Hunter. 1993. "Anatomical Mechanisms Explaining Damage to Pacemaker Leads, Defibrillator Leads, and Failure of Central Venous Catheters Adjacent to the Sternoclavicular Joint." *Pacing and Clinical Electrophysiology* 16: 445–47.

Mond, H. G., and A. Proclemer. 2011. "The 11th World Survey of Cardiac Pacing and Implantable Cardioverter-Defibrillators: Calendar Year 2009: A World Society of Arrhythmia's Project." *Pacing and Clinical Electrophysiology* 34 (8): 1013–27.

Moss, A. J., W. J. Hall, D. S. Cannom, H. Klein, M. W. Brown, J. P. Daubert, N. A. Estes, E. Foster, H. Greenberg, S. L. Higgins, M. A. Pfeffer, S. D. Solomon, D. Wilber, and W. Zareba. 2009. "Cardiac-Resynchronization Therapy for the Prevention of Heart-Failure Events." *The New England Journal of Medicine* 361(14): 1329–38.

Nery, P. B., R. Fernandes, G. M. Nair, G. L. Sumner, C. S. Ribas, S. M. Menon, X. Wang, A. D. Krahn, C. A. Morillo, S. J. Connolly, and J.

S. Healey. 2010. "Device-Related Infection among Patients with Pacemakers and Implantable Defibrillators: Incidence, Risk Factors, and Consequences." *Journal of Cardiovascular Electrophysiology* 21 (7): 786–90.

Noseworthy, P. A., I. Lashevsky, P. Dorian, M. Greene, S. Cvitkovic, and D. Newman. 2004. "Feasibility of Implantable Cardioverter Defibrillator Use in Elderly Patients: A Case Series of Octogenarians." *Pacing and Clinical Electrophysiology* 27: 373–78.

Oginosawa, Y., H. Abe, and Y. Nakashima. 2002. "The Incidence and Risk Factors for Venous Obstruction after Implantation of Transvenous Pacing Leads." *Pacing and Clinical Electrophysiology* 25: 1605–11.

O'Mahony, D. 1995. "Pathophysiology of Carotid Sinus Hypersensitivity in Elderly Patients." *Lancet* 346: 950–52.

Ong, J. J. C., P. C. Hsu, L. Lin, A. Yu, R. M. Kass, C. T. Peter, and C. D. Swerdlow. 1995. "Arrhythmias after Cardioverter-Defibrillator Implantation: Comparison of Epicardial and

Transvenous Systems." *American Journal of Cardiology* 75 (2): 137–40.

Parsonnet, V., A. D. Bernstein, and B. Lindsay. 1989. "Pacemaker-Implantation Complication Rates: An Analysis of Some Contributing Factors." *Journal of the American College of Cardiology* 13 (4): 917–21.

Pedersen, S. S., S. F. Sears, M. M. Burg, and K. C. van den Broek. 2009. "Does ICD Indication Affect Quality of Life and Levels of Distress?" *Pacing and Clinical Electrophysiology* 32: 153–56.

Prudente, L. A., J. Reigle, C. Bourguignon, D. E. Haines, and J. P. DiMarco. 2006. "Psychological Indices and Phantom Shocks in Patients with ICD." *Journal of Interventional Cardiac Electrophysiology* 15: 185–90.

Reynolds, M. R., D. J. Cohen, A. D. Kugelmass, P. P. Brown, E. R. Becker, S. D. Culler, and A. W. Simon. 2006. "The Frequency and Incremental Cost of Major Complications among Medicare Beneficiaries Receiving Implantable Cardioverter-Defibrillators." *Journal of the American College of Cardiology* 47 (12): 2493–97.

Rozmus, G., J. P. Daubert, D. T. Huang, S. Rosero, B. Hall, and C. Francis. 2005. "Venous Thrombosis and Stenosis after Implantation of Pacemakers and Defibrillators." *Journal of Interventional Cardiac Electrophysiology* 13: 9–19.

Santangeli, P., D. S. Frankel, R. Tung, M. Vaseghi, W. H. Sauer, W. S. Tzou, N. Mathuria, S. Nakahara, T. M. Dickfeldt, D. Lakkireddy, T. J. Bunch, L. Di Biase, A. Natale, V. Tholakanahalli, U. B. Tedrow, S. Kumar, W. G. Stevenson, P. Della Bella, K. Shivkumar, F. E. Marchlinski, D. J. Callans. 2017. "Early Mortality After Catheter Ablation of Ventricular Tachycardia in Patients With Structural Heart Disease." *Journal of the American College of Cardiology* 69 (17): 2105-15.

Schulza, N., K. Puschelb, and E. E. Turkc. 2009. "Fatal Complications of Pacemaker and Implantable Cardioverter Defibrillator Implantation: Medical Malpractice?" *Interactive Cardiovascular and Thoracic Surgery* 8: 444–48.

Sears, S. F., and J. B. Conti. 2002. "Quality of Life and Psychological Functioning of ICD Patients." *Heart* 87: 488–93.

Sears, S. F., J. B. Shea, J. B. Conti. 2005. "How to Respond to an Implantable Cardioverter-Defibrillator Shock." *Circulation* 111: e380–82.

Stevenson, R., D. Lugg, R. Gray, D. Hollis, M. Stoner, and J. L. Williams. 2012. "Pacemaker Implantation in the Extreme Elderly." *Journal of Interventional Cardiac Electrophysiology* 33 (1): 51–58.

Tarakji, K. G., E. J. Chan, D. J. Cantillon, A. L. Doonan, T. Hu, S. Schmitt, T. G. Fraser, A. Kim, S. M. Gordon, and B. L. Wilkoff. 2010. "Cardiac Implantable Electronic Device Infections: Presentation, Management, and Patient Outcomes." *Heart Rhythm* 7 (8): 1043–47.

van den Broek, K. C., M. Habibovic, and S. S. Pedersen. 2010. "Emotional Distress in Partners of Patients with an Implantable Cardioverter Defibrillator: A Systematic Review and Recommendations for Future Research." *Pacing and Clinical Electrophysiology* 33: 1442–50.

van Rees J. B., M. K. de Bie, J. Thijssen, C. J. W. Borleffs, M. J. Schalij, and L. van Erven. 2011. "Implantation-Related Complications of Implantable Cardioverter-Defibrillators and Cardiac Resynchronization Therapy Devices." *Journal of the American College of Cardiology* 58 (10): 995–1000.

van Rooden, C. J., S. G. Molhoek, F. R. Rosendaal, M. J. Schalij, A. E. Meinders, and M. V. Huisman. 2004. "Incidence and Risk Factors of Early Venous Thrombosis Associated with Permanent Pacemaker Leads." *Journal of Cardiovascular Electrophysiology* 15: 1258–62.

Wiegand, U. K. H., D. LeJeune, F. Boguschewski, H. Bonnemeier, F. Eberhardt, H. Schunkert, and F. Bode. "Pocket Hematoma after Pacemaker or Implantable Cardioverter Defibrillator Surgery: Influence of Patient Morbidity, Operation Strategy, and Perioperative Antiplatelet/Anticoagulation Therapy." *CHEST* 126 (4): 1177–86.

Wilkoff, B. L. 2007. "How to Treat and Identify Device Infections." *Heart Rhythm* 4: 1467–70.

Worley, S. J., D. C. Gohn, R. W. Pulliam, M. A. Raifsnider, B. Ebersole, and J. Tuzi. "Subclavian Venoplasty by the Implanting Physicians in 373 Patients over 11 Years." *Heart Rhythm* 8 (4): 526–33.

Writing Committee to Revise the ACC/AHA/NASPE 2002 Guideline Update for Implantation of Cardiac Pacemakers and Antiarrhythmia Devices. 2008. "ACC/AHA/HRS 2008 Guidelines for Device-Based Therapy of Cardiac Rhythm Abnormalities: A Report of the American College of Cardiology/American Heart Association Task Force on Practice Guidelines." *Journal of the American College of Cardiology* 51 (21): e1–62.

Yu, C. M., J. Y. S. Chan, Q. Zhang, R. Omar, G. W. K. Yip, A. Hussin, F. Fang, K. H. Lam, H. C. K. Chan, and J. W. H. Fung. 2009. "Biventricular Pacing in Patients with Bradycardia and Normal Ejection Fraction." *The New England Journal of Medicine* 361 (22): 2123–34.

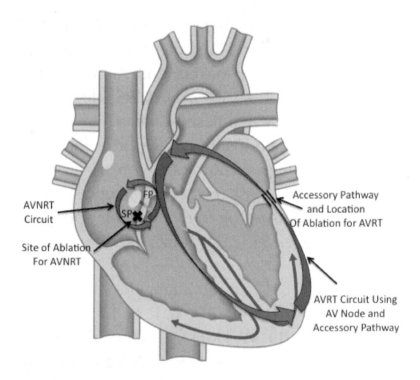

AVNRT
Circuit

Site of Ablation
For AVNRT

FP

SP

Accessory Pathway
and Location
Of Ablation for AVRT

AVRT Circuit Using
AV Node and
Accessory Pathway

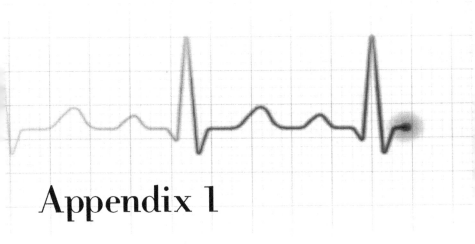

Appendix 1

Atrioventricular Nodal Reentrant Tachycardia (AVNRT) versus Atrioventricular Reentrant Tachycardia (AVRT). In patients with dual AV node physiology, AVNRT occurs when a normal electrical impulse traverses from the atria to the ventricles using the slower AV node pathway (SP) and then immediately sends an electrical signal back up to the atria from the ventricles via the faster AV node pathway (FP). There are several different types of AVNRT, but all types can be treated by performing an ablation (at site labeled X) of the slow AV-node pathway, leaving the fast AV-node pathway intact. In AVRT, a normal electrical impulse traverses from the atrium to the ventricles via the AV node (via the FP) and this impulse is immediately sent back to the atrium via the accessory pathway. The most common location of an accessory pathway (left lateral atrium) and site of ablation (requiring transeptal puncture) is shown.

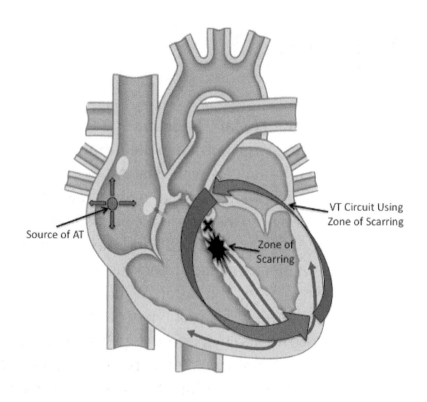

Source of AT

VT Circuit Using
Zone of Scarring

Zone of
Scarring

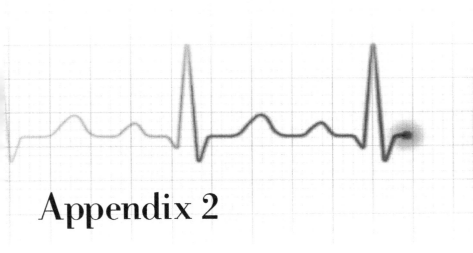

Appendix 2

Atrial Tachycardia (AT) versus Ventricular Tachycardia (VT). Atrial tachycardia (AT) is an SVT caused by an abnormal focus (or cluster) of cells in the top chamber of the heart (left or right atria) that fires irregularly and randomly. AT is generally a nonfatal arrhythmia and can be helped with medications or ablated by targeting the source (or origin) of the AT with ablation. VT may be fatal and is most commonly caused by coronary artery disease (CAD) that leads to scarring of the heart muscle. This scar creates a "circuit" that can cause VT to occur. Ablation of this kind of VT is performed by eradicating pathways (shown by X in this example) that can support the VT circuit. CAD can cause scarring throughout the heart muscle and curing this type of VT may not be possible; this is why medications are usually given before considering ablation. Talk to your doctor about the type of VT you may have.

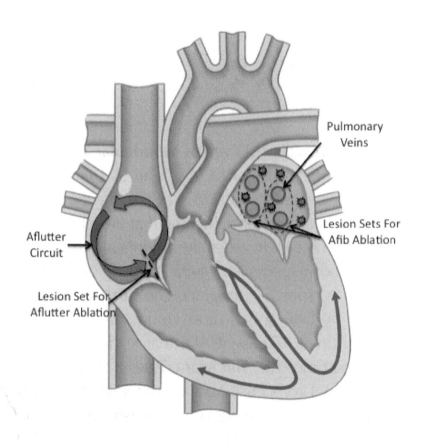

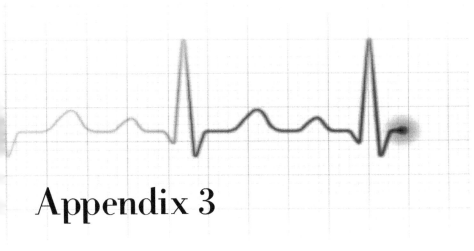

Appendix 3

Atrial Flutter versus Atrial Fibrillation. The figure shows the circuit for typical right atrial flutter and the corresponding line of ablation that may cure this typical atrial flutter. It must be noted that there are atypical atrial flutters that may have vastly different circuits and more complicated ablations. The figure also shows the pulmonary veins in the left atrium; the "triggers" for atrial fibrillation lie within these pulmonary veins. The complicated ablation for atrial fibrillation involves crossing over from the right side to the left side of the heart to perform ablation that electrically isolates the pulmonary veins from the rest of the left atrium. Many patients can have both atrial flutter and fibrillation.

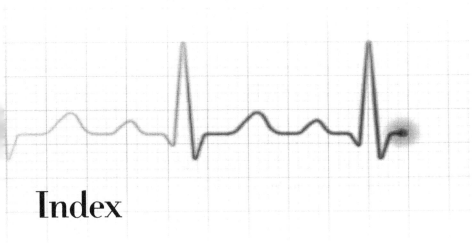

Index

About the Author

Jeffrey L. Williams, MD, MS, FACC, FHRS, CPE, is board certified in internal medicine, cardiovascular disease, and clinical cardiac electrophysiology and is currently a codirector of the Heart Rhythm Center and an Assistant Quality and Medical Informatics Officer at Lakeland Regional Health System. He double majored in biomedical and electrical engineering at Vanderbilt University and then obtained his master's degree in bioengineering from the University of Pittsburgh, where he was awarded a Keck Fellowship for graduate school. Earning his medical degree from Drexel University in Philadelphia, Dr. Williams then went on to complete five years of fellowship training in both cardiovascular disease and clinical cardiac electrophysiology at the University of Pittsburgh Medical Center. Possessing extensive knowledge and a unique background in both engineering and cardiology, Williams has earned numerous accolades within academic and clinical settings, including awards from both the American College of Cardiology Foundation and the National Institutes of Health. Dr. Williams came to Lakeland Regional Health after starting and directing the only community hospital–based Heart Rhythm Center in the United States (2008–2015, The Good Samaritan Hospital) that published outcomes for pacemaker and defibrillator implantations as well as safety and efficacy of high-frequency jet ventilation during electrophysiology studies with ablations. He was elected governor of the Pennsylvania Chapter of the American College of Cardiology in 2015.

48517228R00127

Made in the USA
Columbia, SC
12 January 2019